The Concise Light on Yoga

The Concise Light on Yoga

Yoga Dipika

B. K. S. IYENGAR

Foreword by Yehudi Menuhin

Schocken Books · New York

First American edition published by Schocken Books 1982
10 9 8 7 6 5 4 3 2 1 82 83 84 85

Published by agreement with George Allen & Unwin Ltd., London

Library of Congress Cataloging in Publication Data

Iyengar, B. K. S., 1918–
The concise light on yoga.
Adaptation of: Light on yoga.
Includes index.
1. Yoga, Hatha. I. Iyengar, B.K.S., 1918–
Light on yoga. II. Title.
RA781.7.I937 613.7'046 82-5473 AACR2

Manufactured in the United States of America
ISBN 0-8052-3831-X (hardback)
0-8052-0723-6 (spiralbound)

Dedicated to my Revered Guruji

Sāmkya-yoga-Śikhāmaṇi; Veda-kesari; Vedāntavāgīśa; Nyāyāchārya; Mīmāmsa-ratna; Mīmāmsa-thīrtha

Professor, Śrīmān, T. Krishnamāchārya of Mysore (South India), India

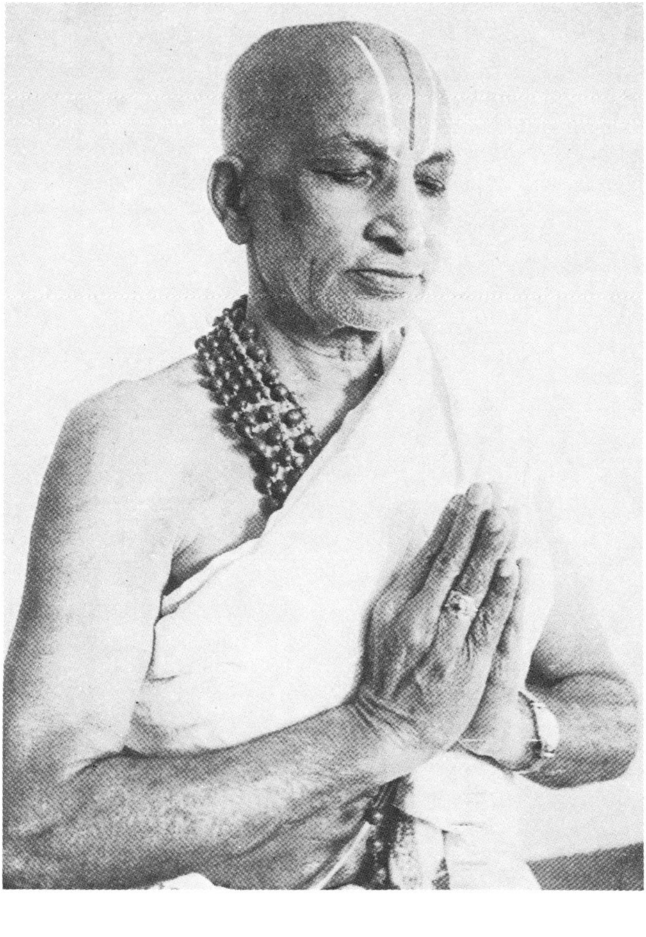

PRAYER

'I bow before the noblest of sages, Patañjali, who brought serenity of mind by his work on yoga, clarity of speech by his work on grammar and purity of body by his work on medicine.'

'I salute Ādīśvara (the Primeval Lord Śiva) who taught first the science of Haṭha Yoga – a science that stands out as a ladder for those who wish to scale the heights of Rāja Yoga.'

Foreword by Yehudi Menuhin

The practice of Yoga induces a primary sense of measure and proportion. Reduced to our own body, our first instrument, we learn to play it, drawing from it maximum resonance and harmony. With unflagging patience we refine and animate every cell as we return daily to the attack, unlocking and liberating capacities otherwise condemned to frustration and death.

Each unfulfilled area of tissue and nerve, of brain or lung, is a challenge to our will and integrity, or otherwise a source of frustration and death. Whoever has had the privilege of receiving Mr Iyengar's attention, or of witnessing the precision, refinement and beauty of his art, is introduced to that vision of perfection and innocence which is man as first created – unarmed, unashamed, son of God, lord of creation – in the Garden of Eden. The tree of knowledge has indeed yielded much fruit of great variety, sweet, poisonous, bitter, wholesome according to our use of it. But is it not more imperative than ever that we cultivate the tree, that we nourish its roots?

The practice of Yoga over the past thirty years has convinced me that most of our fundamental attitudes to life have their physical counter-parts in the body. Thus comparison and criticism must begin with the alignment of our own left and right sides to a degree at which even finer adjustments are feasible: or strength of will may cause us to start by stretching the body from the toes to the top of the head in defiance of gravity. Impetus and ambition might begin with the sense of weight and speed that comes with free-swinging limbs, instead of the control of prolonged balance on foot, feet or hands, which gives poise. Tenacity is gained by stretching in various Yoga postures for minutes at a time, while calmness comes with quiet, consistent breathing and the expansion of the lungs. Continuity and a sense of the universal come with the knowledge of the inevitable alternation of tension and relaxation in eternal rhythms of which each inhalation and exhalation constitutes one cycle, wave or vibration among the countless myriads which are the universe.

What is the alternative? Thwarted, warped people condemning the order of things, cripples criticising the upright, autocrats slumped in expectant coronary attitudes, the tragic spectacle of people working out their own imbalance and frustration on others.

Yoga, as practised by Mr Iyengar, is the dedicated votive offering of a man who brings himself to the altar, alone and clean in body and mind, focussed in attention and will, offering in simplicity and innocence not a burnt sacrifice, but simply himself raised to his own highest potential.

It is a technique ideally suited to prevent physical and mental illness and to protect the body generally, developing an inevitable sense of self-reliance and assurance. By its very nature it is inextricably associated with universal laws: respect for life, truth, and patience are all indispensable factors in the drawing of a quiet breath, in calmness of mind and firmness of will.

In this lie the moral virtues inherent in Yoga. For these reasons it demands a complete and total effort, involving and forming the whole human being. No mechanical repetition is involved and no lip-service as in the case of good resolutions or formal prayers. By its very nature it is each time and every moment a living act.

Mr Iyengar's *Light on Yoga* has, since it was first published fourteen years ago, enabled many to follow his example and become teachers to carry on his work. I was glad at the time to share in its presentation and I welcome this new concise edition equally enthusiastically. It will bring the basic art of Yoga to a much wider audience and will enable it to be practised at the very highest level.

London, 1980

Preface

It is only thanks to the persistent encouragement of my devoted friends and pupils that this book is now achieved – for alone I would have repeatedly faltered not only because of my inadequate command of the English language but because I would have lost heart without their buoyant support and assurance.

Yoga is a timeless pragmatic science evolved over thousands of years dealing with the physical, moral, mental and spiritual well-being of man as a whole.

The first book to systematise this practice was the classic treatise the *Yoga Sutras* (or Aphorisms) of Patañjali dating from 200BC. Unfortunately most of the books published on Yoga in our day have been unworthy of both the subject and its first great exponent, as they are superficial, popular and at times misleading. I have even been asked by their readers whether I can drink acid, chew glass, walk through fire, make myself invisible or perform other magical acts. Scholarly and reliable expositions of the religious and philosophical texts already exist in most languages – but the practice of an art is more difficult to communicate than a purely literary or philosophical concept.

The title of this book is *The Concise Light on Yoga*. Based upon my *Light on Yoga*, which describes *simply* but in great detail the āsanas (postures) and prāṇāyāmas (breathing disciplines), this new book provides a comprehensive introduction to yoga. It describes the techniques for 57 āsanas with the aid of 147 photographs and it also covers prāṇāyāma with the aid of another four photographs.

The Western reader may be surprised at the recurring reference to the Universal Spirit, to mythology and even to philosophical and moral principles. He must not forget that in ancient times all the higher achievements of man, in knowledge, art and power, were part of religion and were assumed to belong to God and to His priestly servants on earth. The Catholic Pope is the last such embodiment of divine knowledge and power in the West. But formerly, even in the Western world, music, painting, architecture, philosophy and medicine, as well as wars, were always in the service of God. It is only very recently in India that these arts and sciences have begun to shake off the Divine – but with due respect, for the emancipation of man's will, as distinct from the Divine will, we in India continue to value the purity of purpose, the humility of discipline and the selflessness that are the legacy of our long bondage to God. I consider it important as well as interesting that the reader should know the origin of āsanas, and I have, therefore, included legends handed down by practising yogis and sages.

All the ancient commentaries on yoga have stressed that it is essential to work under the direction of a GURU (Master), and although my experience proves the wisdom of this rule, I have endeavoured with all humility in this book to guide the reader – both teacher and student – to a correct and safe method of mastering these āsanas and prāṇāyāmas.

In the Appendix, I have introduced a 35 weeks' course for the intense practitioner, grouping the āsanas stage by stage according to their structure.

Study in detail the hints and cautions before attempting the āsana and prāṇāyāma techniques.

I am sincerely grateful to my esteemed friend and pupil Mr Yehudi Menuhin for his foreword and immeasurable support.

I am indebted to my pupil Mr B. I. Taraporewala for his collaboration in the preparation of this book.

I thank Unwin Paperbacks for their gesture in publishing this abridged version and presenting my work to a world-wide public.

I express my sincere gratitude to Messrs G. G. Welling of Poona (India), for their personal supervision and interest in taking innumerable photographs for me and for placing the resources of their studio at my disposal.

B. K. S. IYENGAR

Contents

Part I

What is Yoga?

What is Yoga?

The word Yoga is derived from the Sanskrit root yuj meaning to bind, join, attach and yoke, to direct and concentrate one's attention on, to use and apply. It also means union or communion. It is the true union of our will with the will of God. 'It thus means,' says Mahadev Desai in his introduction to the *Gita according to Gandhi*, 'the yoking of all the powers of body, mind and soul to God; it means the disciplining of the intellect, the mind, the emotions, the will, which that Yoga presupposes; it means a poise of the soul which enables one to look at life in all its aspects evenly.'

Yoga is one of the six orthodox systems of Indian philosophy. It was collated, co-ordinated and systematised by Patañjali in his classical work, the *Yoga Sutras,* which consists of 185 terse aphorisms. In Indian thought, everything is permeated by the Supreme Universal Spirit (Paramātmā or God) of which the individual human spirit (jīvātmā) is a part. The system of yoga is so called because it teaches the means by which the jīvātmā can be united to, or be in communion with the Paramātmā, and so secure liberation (mokṣa).

One who follows the path of Yoga is a yogi or yogin.

In the sixth chapter of the *Bhagavad Gītā,* which is the most important authority on Yoga philosophy, Śri Krishna explains to Arjuna the meaning of Yoga as a deliverance from contact with pain and sorrow. It is said:

'When his mind, intellect and self (ahaṁkāra) are under control, freed from restless desire, so that they rest in the spirit within, a man becomes a Yukta – one in communion with God. A lamp does not flicker in a place where no winds blow; so it is with a yogi, who controls his mind, intellect and self, being absorbed in the spirit within him. When the restlessness of the mind, intellect and self is stilled through the practice of Yoga, the yogi by the grace of the Spirit within himself finds fulfilment. Then he knows the joy eternal which is beyond the pale of the senses which his reason cannot grasp. He abides in this reality and moves not therefrom. He has found the treasure above all others. There is nothing higher than this. He who has achieved it, shall not be moved by the greatest sorrow. This is the real meaning of Yoga – a deliverance from contact with pain and sorrow.'

As a well cut diamond has many facets, each reflecting a different colour of light, so does the word yoga, each facet reflecting a different shade of meaning and revealing different aspects of the entire range of human endeavour to win inner peace and happiness.

The *Bhagavad Gītā* also gives other explanations of the term yoga and lays stress upon Karma Yoga (Yoga by action). It is said: 'Work alone is your privilege, never the fruits thereof. Never let the fruits of action be your motive; and never cease to work. Work in the name of the Lord, abandoning selfish desires. Be not affected by success or failure. This equipoise is called Yoga.'

Yoga has also been described as wisdom in work or skilful living amongst activities with harmony and moderation.
'Yoga is not for him who gorges too much, nor for him who starves himself. It is not for him who sleeps too much, nor for him who stays awake. By moderation in eating and in resting, by regulation in working and by concordance in sleeping and waking, Yoga destroys all pain and sorrow.'

The *Kaṭhopanishad* describes Yoga thus: 'When the senses are stilled, when the mind is at rest, when the intellect wavers not – then, say the wise, is reached the highest stage. This steady control of the senses and mind has been defined as Yoga. He who attains it is free from delusion.'

In the second aphorism of the first chapter of the *Yoga Sutras*, Patañjali describes Yoga as '*chitta vṛtti nirodhah*'. This may be translated as the restraint (nirodhah) of mental (chitta) modifications (vṛtti) or as suppression (nirodhah) of the fluctuations (vṛtti) of consciousness (chitta). The word chitta denotes the mind in its total or collective sense as being composed of three categories: (a) mind (manas, that is, the individual mind having the power and faculty of attention, selection and rejection; it is the oscillating indecisive faculty of the mind); (b) intelligence or reason (buddhi, that is, the decisive state which determines the distinction between things) and (c) ego (ahaṁkāra, literally the I-maker, the state which ascertains that 'I know').

The word vṛtti is derived from the Sanskrit root vṛt meaning to turn, to revolve, to roll on. It thus means course of action, behaviour, mode of being, condition or mental state. Yoga is the method by which the restless mind is calmed and the energy directed into constructive channels. As a mighty river which when properly harnessed by dams and canals, creates a vast reservoir of water, prevents famine and provides abundant power for industry; so also the mind, when controlled, provides a reservoir of peace and generates abundant energy for human uplift.

The problem of controlling the mind is not capable of easy solution, as borne out by the following dialogue in the sixth chapter of the *Bhagavad Gītā*. Arjuna asks Śri Krishna:

'Krishna, you have told me of Yoga as a communion with Brahman (the Universal Spirit), which is ever one. But how can this be permanent, since the mind is so restless and inconsistent? The mind is impetuous and stubborn, strong and wilful, as difficult to harness as the wind.' Śri Krishna replies: 'Undoubtedly, the mind is restless and hard to control. But it can be trained by constant practice (abhyāsa) and by freedom from desire (vairāgya). A man who cannot control his mind will find it difficult to attain this divine communion; but the self-controlled man can attain it if he tries hard and directs his energy by the right means.'

THE STAGES OF YOGA

The right means are just as important as the end in view. Patañjali enumerates these means as the eight limbs or stages of Yoga for the quest of the soul. They are:

1. Yama (universal moral commandments); 2. Niyama

(self purification by discipline); 3. Asana (posture); 4. Prāṇāyāma (rhythmic control of the breath); 5. Pratyāhāra (withdrawal and emancipation of the mind from the domination of the senses and exterior objects); 6. Dhāraṇa (concentration); 7. Dhyāna (meditation) and 8. Samādhi (a state of super-consciousness brought about by profound meditation, in which the individual aspirant (sādhaka) becomes one with the object of his meditation – Paramātmā or the Universal Spirit).

Yama and Niyama control the yogi's passions and emotions and keep him in harmony with his fellow man. Ásanas keep the body healthy and strong and in harmony with nature. Finally, the yogi becomes free of body consciousness. He conquers the body and renders it a fit vehicle for the soul. The first three stages are the outward quests (bahiranga sādhanā).

The next two stages, Prāṇāyāma and Pratyāhāra, teach the aspirant to regulate the breathing, and thereby control the mind. This helps to free the senses from the thraldom of the objects of desire. These two stages of Yoga are known as the inner quests (antaranga sādhanā).

Dhāranā, Dhyāna and Samādhi take the yogi into the innermost recesses of his soul. The yogi does not look heavenward to find God. He knows that HE is within, being known as the Antarātmā (the Inner Self). The last three stages keep him in harmony with himself and his Maker. These stages are called antarātmā sādhanā, the quest of the soul.

By profound meditation, the knower, the knowledge and the known become one. The seer, the sight and the seen have no separate existence from each other. It is like a great musician becoming one with his instrument and the music that comes from it. Then, the yogi stands in his own nature and realises his self (Ātman), the part of the Supreme Soul within himself.

There are different paths (mārgas) by which a man travels to his Maker. The active man finds realisation through Karma Mārga, in which a man realises his own divinity through work and duty. The emotional man finds it through

Bhakti Mārga, where there is realisation through devotion to and love of a personal God. The intellectual man pursues Jñāna, Mārga, where realisation comes through knowledge. The meditative or reflective man follows Yoga Mārga, and realises his own divinity through control of the mind.

Happy is the man who knows how to distinguish the real from the unreal, the eternal from the transient and the good from the pleasant by his discrimination and wisdom. Twice blessed is he who knows true love and can love all God's creatures. He who works selflessly for the welfare of others with love in his heart is thrice blessed. But the man who combines within his mortal frame knowledge, love and selfless service is holy and becomes a place of pilgrimage, like the confluence of the rivers Gangā, Saraswatī and Jamunā. Those who meet him become calm and purified.

Mind is the king of the senses. One who has conquered his mind, senses, passions, thought and reason is a king among men. He is fit for Rāja Yoga, the royal union with the Universal Spirit. He has Inner Light.

He who has conquered his mind is Rāja Yogi. The word rāja means a king. The expression Rāja Yoga implies a complete mastery of the Self. Though Patañjali explains the ways to control the mind, he nowhere states in his aphorisms that this science is Rāja Yoga, but calls it Aṣṭāṅga Yoga or the eight stages (limbs) of Yoga. As it implies complete mastery of the self one may call it the science of Rāja Yoga.

Swātmārāma, the author of the *Hatha Yoga Pradīpikā* (haṭha=force or determined effort) called the same path Haṭha Yoga because it demanded rigorous discipline.

It is generally believed that Rāja Yoga and Haṭha Yoga are entirely distinct, different and opposed to each other, that the *Yoga Sutras* of Patañjāli deal with Spiritual discipline and that the *Haṭha Yoga Pradīpikā* of Swātmārāma deals solely with physical discipline. It is not so, for Haṭha Yoga and Rāja Yoga complement each other and form a single approach towards Liberation. As a mountaineer needs ladders, ropes and crampons as well as physical fitness and discipline to climb the icy peaks of the Himālayas, so does the Yoga aspirant need the knowledge and discipline of the Haṭha

Yoga of Swātmārāma to reach the heights of Rāja Yoga dealt with by Patañjali.

This path of Yoga is the fountain for the other three paths. It brings calmness and tranquillity and prepares the mind for absolute unqualified self-surrender to God, in which all these four paths merge into one.

Chitta Vṛtti (Causes for the Modification of the Mind)

In his *Yoga Sutras* Patañjali lists five classes of chitta vṛtti which create pleasure and pain. These are:

1. Pramāṇa (a standard or ideal), by which things or values are measured by the mind or known, which men accept upon (a) direct evidence such as perception (pratyakṣa), (b) inference (anumāna) and (c) testimony or the word of an acceptable authority when the source of knowledge has been checked as reliable and trustworthy (āgama).

2. Viparyaya (a mistaken view which is observed to be such after study). A faulty medical diagnosis based on wrong hypotheses, or the formerly held theory in astronomy that the Sun rotates round the Earth, are examples of viparyaya.

3. Vikalpa (fancy or imagination, resting merely on verbal expression without any factual basis). A beggar may feel happy when he imagines himself spending millions. A rich miser, on the other hand, may starve himself in the belief that he is poor.

4. Nidrā (sleep), where there is the absence of ideas and experiences. When a man is sleeping soundly, he does not recall his name, family or status, his knowledge or wisdom, or even his own existence. When a man forgets himself in sleep, he wakes up refreshed. But, if a disturbing thought creeps into his mind when he is dropping off, he will not rest properly.

5. Smṛti (memory, the holding fast of the impressions of objects that one has experienced). There are people who live

in their past experiences, even though the past is beyond recall. Their sad or happy memories keep them chained to the past and they cannot break their fetters.

Patañjali enumerates five causes of chitta vṛtti creating pain (kleśa). These are:

1. Avidyā (ignorance or nescience); (2) asmitā (the feeling of individuality which limits a person and distinguishes him from a group and which may be physical, mental, intellectual or emotional); (3) rāga (attachment or passion); (4) dveśa (aversion or revulsion) and (5) abhiniveśa (love of or thirst for life, the instinctive clinging to worldly life and bodily enjoyment and the fear that one may be cut off from all this by death). These causes of pain remain submerged in the mind of the sādhaka (the aspirant or seeker). They are like icebergs barely showing their heads in the polar seas. So long as they are not studiously controlled and eradicated, there can be no peace. The yogi learns to forget the past and takes no thought for the morrow. He lives in the eternal present.

As a breeze ruffles the surface of a lake and distorts the images reflected therein, so also the chitta vṛtti disturb the peace of the mind. The still waters of a lake reflect the beauty around it. When the mind is still, the beauty of the Self is seen reflected in it. The yogi stills his mind by constant study and by freeing himself from desires. The eight stages of Yoga teach him the way.

Chitta Vikṣepa (Distractions and Obstacles)

The distractions and obstacles which hinder the aspirant's practice of Yoga are:

1 Vyādhi – sickness which disturbs the physical equilibrium
2 Styāna – languor or lack of mental disposition for work
3 Saṁśaya – doubt or indecision
4 Pramāda – indifference or insensibility
5 Ālasya – laziness

6 Avirati – sensuality, the rousing of desire when sensory objects possess the mind
7 Bhrānti Darśana – false or invalid knowledge, or illusion
8 Alabdha Bhūmikatva – failure to attain continuity of thought or concentration so that reality cannot be seen
9 Anavasthitattva – instability in holding on to concentration which has been attained after long practice.

There are, however, four more distractions: (1) duḥkha – pain or misery, (2) daurmanasya – despair, (3) aṅgamejayatva – unsteadiness of the body and (4) ṣvāsa-praśvāsa – unsteady respiration.

To win a battle, a general surveys the terrain and the enemy and plans counter-measures. In a similar way the Yogi plans the conquest of the Self.

Vyādhi: It will be noticed that the very first obstacle is ill-health or sickness. To the yogi his body is the prime instrument of attainment. If his vehicle breaks down, the traveller cannot go far. If the body is broken by ill-health, the aspirant can achieve little. Physical health is important for mental development, as normally the mind functions through the nervous system. When the body is sick or the nervous system is affected, the mind becomes restless or dull and inert and concentration or meditation become impossible.

Styāna: A person suffering from languor has no goal, no path to follow and no enthusiasm. His mind and intellect become dull due to inactivity and their faculties rust. Constant flow keeps a mountain stream pure, but water in a ditch stagnates and nothing good can flourish in it. A listless person is like a living corpse for he can concentrate on nothing.

Samśaya: The unwise, the faithless and the doubter destroy themselves. How can they enjoy this world or the next or have any happiness? The seeker should have faith in himself and his master. He should have faith that God is ever by his side and that no evil can touch him. As faith springs up in the heart it dries out lust, ill-will, mental sloth, spiritual pride and doubt, and the heart free from these hindrances becomes serene and untroubled.

Pramāda: A person suffering from pramāda is full of self-importance, lacks any humility and believes that he alone is wise. No doubt he knows what is right or wrong, but he persists in his indifference to the right and chooses what is pleasant. To gratify his selfish passions and dreams of personal glory, he will deliberately and without scruple sacrifice everyone who stands in his way. Such a person is blind of God's glory and deaf to His words.

Ālasya: To remove the obstacle of laziness, unflagging enthusiasm (vīrya) is needed. The attitude of the aspirant is like that of a lover ever yearning to meet the beloved but never giving way to despair. Hope should be his shield and courage his sword. He should be free from hate and sorrow. With faith and enthusiasm he should overcome the inertia of the body and the mind.

Avirati: This is the tremendous craving for sensory objects after they have been consciously abandoned, which is so hard to restrain. Without being attached to the objects of sense, the yogi learns to enjoy them with the aid of the senses which are completely under his control. By the practice of pratyāhāra he wins freedom from attachment and emancipation from desire and becomes content and tranquil.

Bhrānti Darśana: A person afflicted by false knowledge suffers from delusion and believes that he alone has seen the true Light. He has a powerful intellect but lacks humility and makes a show of wisdom. By remaining in the company of great souls and through their guidance he sets his foot firmly on the right path and overcomes his weakness.

Alabdha Bhūmikatva: As a mountain climber fails to reach the summit for lack of stamina, so also a person who cannot overcome the inability to concentrate is unable to seek reality. He might have had glimpses of reality but he cannot see clearly. He is like a musician who has heard divine music in a dream, but who is unable to recall it in his waking moments and cannot repeat the dream.

Anavasthitattva: A person affected with anavasthitattva has by hard work come within sight of reality. Happy and proud of his achievements he becomes slack in his practice (sādhanā). He has purity and great power of concentration and has come to the final cross-roads of his quest. Even at this last stage continuous endeavour is essential and he has to pursue the path with infinite patience and determined perseverance and must never show slackness which hampers progress on the path of God realization. He must wait until divine grace descends upon him. It has been said in the *Kaṭhopanisad:* 'The Self is not to be realised by study and instruction, nor by subtlety of intellect, nor by much learning, but only by him who longs for Him, by the one whom He chooses. Verily to such a one the Self reveals His true being.'

To overcome the obstacles and to win unalloyed happiness, Patañjali offered several remedies. The best of these is the fourfold remedy of Maitri (friendliness), Karuṇa (compassion), Mudiṭā (delight) and Upekṣā (disregard).

Maitri is not merely friendliness, but also a feeling of oneness with the object of friendliness (ātmīyatā). A mother feels intense happiness at the success of her children because of ātmīyatā, a feeling of oneness. Patañjali recommends maitri for sukha (happiness or virtue). The yogi cultivates maitri and ātmīyatā for the good and turns enemies into friends, bearing malice towards none.

Karuṇa is not merely showing pity or compassion and shedding tears of despair at the misery (duḥkha) of others. It is compassion coupled with devoted action to relieve the misery of the afflicted. The yogi uses all his resources – physical, economic, mental or moral – to alleviate the pain and suffering of others. He shares his strength with the weak until they become strong. He shares his courage with those that are timid until they become brave by his example. He denies the maxim of the 'survival of the fittest', but makes the weak strong enough to survive. He becomes a shelter to one and all.

Muditā is a feeling of delight at the good work (punya) done by another, even though he may be a rival. Through muditā, the yogi saves himself from much heart-burning by not showing anger, hatred or jealousy for another who has reached the desired goal which he himself has failed to achieve.

Upekṣā: It is not merely a feeling of disdain or contempt for the person who has fallen into vice (apuṇya) or one of indifference or superiority towards him. It is a searching self-examination to find out how one would have behaved when faced with the same temptations. It is also an examination to see how far one is responsible for the state into which the unfortunate one has fallen and the attempt thereafter to put him on the right path. The yogi understands the faults of others by seeing and studying them first in himself. This self-study teaches him to be charitable to all.

The deeper significance of the fourfold remedy of maitri, karuṇa, muditā and upekṣā cannot be felt by an unquiet mind. My experience has led me to conclude that for an ordinary man or woman in any community of the world, the way to achieve a quiet mind is to work with determination on two of the eight stages of Yoga mentioned by Patañjali, namely, āsana and prāṇāyāma.

The mind (manas) and the breath (prāṇa) are intimately connected and the activity or the cessation of activity of one affects the other. Hence Patañjali recommended prāṇāyāma (rhythmic breath control) for achieving mental equipoise and inner peace.

Śiṣya and Guru (A Pupil and a Master)

The *Śiva Samhitā* divides sādhakas (pupils or aspirants) into four classes. They are (1) mṛdu (feeble), (2) madhyama (average), (3) adhimātra (superior) and (4) adhimātratama (the supreme one). The last, the highest, is alone able to cross beyond the ocean of the manifest world.

The feeble seekers are those who lack enthusiasm, criticise

their teachers, are rapacious, inclined to bad action, eat much, are in the power of women, unstable, cowardly, ill, dependent, speak harshly, have weak characters and lack virility. The Guru (Teacher or Master) guides such seekers in the path of Mantra Yoga only. With much effort, the sādhaka can reach enlightenment in twelve years. (The word mantra is derived from the root 'man', meaning to think. Mantra thus means a sacred thought or prayer to be repeated with full understanding of its meaning. It takes a long time, perhaps years, for a mantra to take firm root in the mind of a feeble sādhaka and still longer for it to bear fruit.)

Of even mind, capable of bearing hardship, wishing to perfect the work, speaking gently, moderate in all circumstances, such is the average seeker. Recognising these qualities, the Guru teaches him Laya Yoga, which gives liberation. (Laya means devotion, absorption or dissolution.)

Of stable mind, capable of Laya Yoga, virile, independent, noble, merciful, forgiving, truthful, brave, young, respectful, worshipping his teacher, intent on the practice of Yoga, such is a superior seeker. He can reach enlightenment after six years of practice. The Guru instructs this forceful man in Haṭha Yoga.

Of great virility and enthusiasm, good looking, courageous, learned in scriptures, studious, sane in mind, not melancholic, keeping young, regular in food, with his senses under control, free from fear, clean, skilful, generous, helpful to all, firm, intelligent, independent, forgiving, of good character, of gentle speech and worshipping his Guru, such is a supreme seeker, fit for all forms of Yoga. He can reach enlightenment in three years.

Although the *Śiva Samhitā* and the *Haṭha Yoga Pradīpikā* mention the period of time within which success might be achieved, Patañjali nowhere lays down the time required to unite the individual soul with the Divine Universal Soul. According to him abhyāsa (constant and determined practice) and vairāgya (freedom from desires) make the mind calm and tranquil. He defines abhyāsa as effort of long duration, without interruption, performed with devotion, which creates a firm foundation.

The study of Yoga is not like work for a diploma or a university degree by someone desiring favourable results in a stipulated time.

The obstacles, trials and tribulations in the path of Yoga can be removed to a large extent with the help of a Guru. (The syllable gu means darkness and ru means light. He alone is a Guru who removes darkness and brings enlightenment.) The conception of a Guru is deep and significant. He is not an ordinary guide. He is a spiritual teacher who teaches a way of life, and not merely how to earn a livelihood. He transmits knowledge of the Spirit and one who receives such knowledge is a śiṣya, a disciple.

The relationship between a Guru and a śiṣya is a very special one, transcending that between parent and child, husband and wife or friends. A Guru is free from egotism. He devotedly leads his śiṣya towards the ultimate goal without any attraction for fame or gain. He shows the path of God and watches the progress of his disciple, guiding him along that path. He inspires confidence, devotion, discipline, deep understanding and illumination through love. With faith in his pupil, the Guru strains hard to see that he absorbs the teaching. He encourages him to ask question and to know the truth by question and analysis.

A śiṣya should possess the necessary qualifications of higher realisation and development. He must have confidence, devotion and love for his Guru. The perfect examples of the relationship between a Guru and a śiṣya are those of Yama (the God of Death) and Nachiketā in the *Kaṭhopaniṣad* and of Śri Krishna and Arjuna in the *Bhagavad Gītā*. Nachiketā and Arjuna obtained enlightenment through their one-pointed mind, their eagerness and questioning spirit. The śiṣya should hunger for knowledge and have the spirit of humility, perseverance and tenacity of purpose. He should not go to the Guru merely out of curiosity. He should possess śraddhā (dynamic faith) and should not be discouraged if he cannot reach the goal in the time he had expected. It requires tremendous patience to calm the restless mind which is coloured by innumerable past experiences and saṁskāra (the accumulated residue of past thoughts and actions).

Merely listening to the words of the Guru does not enable the śiṣya to absorb the teaching. This is borne out by the story of Indra and Virochana. Indra, the king of Gods, and Virochana, a demon prince, went together to their spiritual preceptor Brahmā to obtain knowledge of the Supreme Self. Both stayed and listened to the same words of their Guru. Indra obtained enlightenment, whereas Virochana did not. Indra's memory was developed by his devotion to the subject taught by the love and faith which he had for his teacher. He had a feeling of oneness with his Guru. These were the reasons for his success. Virochana's memory was developed only through his intellect. He had no devotion either for the subject taught or for his preceptor. He remained what he originally was, an intellectual giant. He returned a doubter. Indra had intellectual humility, while Virochana had intellectual pride and imagined that it was condescending on his part to go to Brahmā. The approach of Indra was devotional while that of Virochana was practical. Virochana was motivated by curiosity and wanted the practical knowledge which he believed would be useful to him later to win power.

The śiṣya should above all treasure love, moderation and humility. Love begets courage, moderation creates abundance and humility generates power. Courage without love is brutish. Abundance without moderation leads to overindulgence and decay. Power without humility breeds arrogance and tyranny. The true śiṣya learns from his Guru about a power which will never leave him as he returns to the Primeval One, the Source of His Being.

Sādhanā (A Key to Freedom)

All the important texts on Yoga lay great emphasis on sādhanā or abhyāsa (constant practice). Sādhanā is not just a theoretical study of Yoga texts. It is a spiritual endeavour. Oil seeds must be pressed to yield oil. Wood must be heated to ignite and bring out the hidden fire within. In the same way, the sādhaka must by constant practice light the divine flame within himself.

'The young, the old, the extremely aged, even the sick and the infirm obtain perfection in Yoga by constant practice.

Success will follow him who practises, not him who practises not. Success in Yoga is not obtained by the mere theoretical reading of sacred texts. Success is not obtained by wearing the dress of a yogi or a sanyāsi (a recluse), nor by talking about it. Constant practice alone is the secret of success. Verily, there is no doubt of this.' – (*Haṭha Yoga Pradīpikā*, chapter 1. verses 64–6.)

'As by learning the alphabet one can, through practice, master all the sciences, so by thoroughly practising first physical training one acquires the knowledge of Truth (Tattva Jñāna), that is the real nature of the human soul as being identical with the Supreme Spirit pervading the Universe.' – (*Gheraṇḍa Saṁhitā*, chapter 1, verse 5.)

It is by the co-ordinated and concentrated efforts of his body, senses, mind, reason and Self that a man obtains the prize of inner peace and fulfils the quest of his soul to meet his Maker. The supreme adventure in a man's life is his journey back to his Creator. To reach the goal he needs well developed and co-ordinated functioning of his body, senses, mind, reason and Self. If the effort is not co-ordinated, he fails in his adventure. In the third valli (chapter) of the first part of the *Kaṭhopaniṣad*, Yama (the God of Death) explains this Yoga to the seeker Nachiketā by way of the parable of the individual in a chariot.

'Know the Ātman (Self) as the Lord in a chariot, reason as the charioteer and mind as the reins. The senses, they say, are the horses, and their objects of desire are the pastures. The Self, when united with the senses and the mind, the wise call the Enjoyer (Bhoktṛ). The undiscriminating can never rein in his mind; his senses are like the vicious horses of a charioteer. The discriminating ever controls his mind; his senses are like disciplined horses. The undiscriminating becomes unmindful, ever impure; he does not reach the goal, wandering from one body to another. The discriminating becomes mindful, ever pure; he reaches the goal and is never reborn. The man who has a discriminating charioteer to rein in his mind reaches the end of the journey – the Supreme Abode of the everlasting Spirit.'

'The senses are more powerful than the objects of desire.

Greater than the senses is the mind, higher than the mind is the reason and superior to reason is He – the Spirit in all. Discipline yourself by the Self and destroy your deceptive enemy in the shape of desire.' (*Bhagavad Gītā,* chapter III, verses 42–3.)

To realise this not only constant practice is demanded but also renunciation. As regards renunciation, the question arises as to what one should renounce. The yogi does not renounce the world, for that would mean renouncing the Creator. The yogi renounces all that takes him away from the Lord. He renounces his own desires, knowing that all inspiration and right action come from the Lord. He renounces those who oppose the work of the Lord, those who spread demonic ideas and who merely talk of moral values but do not practise them.

The yogi does not renounce action. He cuts the bonds that tie himself to his actions by dedicating their fruits either to the Lord or to humanity. He believes that it is his privilege to do his duty and that he has no right to the fruits of his actions.

While others are asleep when duty calls and wake up only to claim their rights, the yogi is fully awake to his duty, but asleep over his rights. Hence it is said that in the night of all beings the disciplined and tranquil man wakes to the light.

Aṣṭāṅga Yoga – The Eight Limbs of Yoga

The *Yoga Sutra* of Patañjali is divided into four chapters or pāda. The first deals with samādhi, the second with the means (sādhanā) to achieve Yoga, the third enumerates the powers (vibhūti) that the yogi comes across in his quest, and the fourth deals with absolution (kaivalya).

Yama

The eight limbs of Yoga are described in the second chapter. The first of these is yama (ethical disciplines) – the great commandments transcending creed, country, age and time. They are: ahimsā (non-violence), satya (truth), asteya (non-stealing), brahmacharya (continence) and aparigraha (non-coveting). These commandments are the rules of morality for society and the individual, which if not obeyed bring chaos, violence, untruth, stealing, dissipation and covetousness. The roots of these evils are the emotions of greed, desire and attachment, which may be mild, medium or excessive. They only bring pain and ignorance. Patañjali strikes at the root of these evils by changing the direction of one's thinking along the five principles of yama.

Ahimsā. The word ahimsā is made up of the particle 'a' meaning 'not' and the noun himsā meaning killing or violence. It is more than a negative command not to kill, for it has a wider positive meaning, love. This love embraces all creation for we are all children of the same Father – the Lord. The yogi believes that to kill or to destroy a thing or being is to insult its Creator. Men either kill for food or to protect themselves from danger. But merely because a man is a vegetarian, it does not necessarily follow that he is non-violent by temperament or that he is a yogi, though a vegetarian diet is a necessity for the practice of yoga. Blood-thirsty tyrants may be vegetarians, but violence is a state of mind, not of diet. It resides in a man's mind and not in the instrument he holds in his hand. One can use a knife to pare fruit or to stab an enemy. The fault is not in the instrument, but in the user.

Men take to violence to protect their own interests – their own bodies, their loved ones, their property or dignity. But a man cannot rely upon himself alone to protect himself or others. The belief that he can do so is wrong. A man must rely upon God, who is the source of all strength. Then he will fear no evil.

Violence arises out of fear, weakness, ignorance or restlessness. To curb it what is most needed is freedom from fear. To gain this freedom, what is required is a change of outlook on life and reorientation of the mind. Violence is bound to decline when men learn to base their faith upon reality and investigation rather than upon ignorance and supposition.

The yogi believes that every creature has as much right to live as he has. He believes that he is born to help others and he looks upon creation with eyes of love. He knows that his life is linked inextricably with that of others and he rejoices if he can help them to be happy. He puts the happiness of others before his own and becomes a source of joy to all who meet him. As parents encourage a baby to walk the first steps, he encourages those more unfortunate than himself and makes them fit for survival.

For a wrong done by others, men demand justice; while for that done by themselves they plead mercy and forgiveness. The yogi on the other hand, believes that for a wrong done by himself, there should be justice, while for that done by another there should be forgiveness. He knows and teaches others how to live. Always striving to perfect himself, he shows them by his love and compassion how to improve themselves.

The yogi opposes the evil in the wrong-doer, but not the wrong-doer. He prescribes penance not punishment for a wrong done. Opposition to evil and love for the wrong-doer can live side by side. A drunkard's wife whilst loving him may still oppose his habit. Opposition without love leads to violence; loving the wrong-doer without opposing the evil in him is folly and leads to misery. The yogi knows that to love a person whilst fighting the evil in him is the right course to follow. The battle is won because he fights it with love. A loving mother will sometimes beat her child to cure it of a bad habit; in the same way a true follower of ahimsā loves his opponent.

Along with ahimsā go abhaya (freedom from fear) and akrodha (freedom from anger). Freedom from fear comes only to those who lead a pure life. The yogi fears none and none need fear him, because he is purified by the study of the Self. Fear grips a man and paralyses him. He is afraid of the future, the unknown and the unseen. He is afraid that he may lose his means of livelihood, wealth or reputation. But the greatest fear is that of death. The yogi knows that he is different from his body, which is a temporary house for his spirit. He sees all beings in the Self and the Self in all beings and therefore he loses all fear. Though the body is subject to sickness, age, decay and death, the spirit remains unaffected. To the yogi death is the sauce that adds zest to life. He has dedicated his mind, his reason and his whole life to the Lord.

When he has linked his entire being to the Lord, what shall he then fear?

There are two types of anger (krodha), one of which debases the mind while the other leads to spiritual growth. The root of the first is pride, which makes one angry when slighted. This prevents the mind from seeing things in perspective and makes one's judgement defective. The yogi, on the other hand, is angry with himself when his mind stoops low or when all his learning and experience fail to stop him from folly. He is stern with himself when he deals with his own faults, but gentle with the faults of others. Gentleness of mind is an attribute of a yogi, whose heart melts at all suffering. In him gentleness for others and firmness for himself go hand in hand, and in his presence all hostilities are given up.

Satya. Satya or truth is the highest rule of conduct or morality. Mahātma Gandhi said: 'Truth is God and God is Truth.' As fire burns impurities and refines gold, so the fire of truth cleanses the yogi and burns up the dross in him.

If the mind thinks thoughts of truth, if the tongue speaks words of truth and if the whole life is based upon truth, then one becomes fit for union with the Infinite. Reality in its fundamental nature is love and truth and expresses itself through these two aspects. The yogi's life must conform strictly to these two facets of Reality. That is why ahimsā, which is essentially based on love, is enjoined. Satya presupposes perfect truthfulness in thought, word and deed. Untruthfulness in any form puts the sādhaka out of harmony with the fundamental law of truth.

Truth is not limited to speech alone. There are four sins of speech: abuse and obscenity, dealing in falsehoods, calumny or telling tales and lastly ridiculing what others hold to be sacred. The tale bearer is more poisonous than a snake. The control of speech leads to the rooting out of malice. When the mind bears malice towards none, it is filled with charity towards all. He who has learnt to control his tongue has attained self-control in a great measure. When such a person speaks he will be heard with respect and attention. His words will be remembered, for they will be good and true.

When one who is established in truth prays with a pure heart, then things he really needs come to him when they are really needed: he does not have to run after them. The man firmly established in truth gets the fruit of his actions without apparently doing anything. God, the source of all truth, supplies his needs and looks after his welfare.

Asteya. The desire to possess and enjoy what another has, drives a person to do evil deeds. From this desire spring the urge to steal and the urge to covet. Asteya (a=not, steya= stealing), or non-stealing includes not only taking what belongs to another without permission, but also using something for a different purpose to that intended, or beyond the time permitted by its owner. It thus includes misappropriation, breach of trust, mismanagement and misuse. The yogi reduces his physical needs to the minimum, believing that if he gathers things he does not really need, he is a thief. While other men crave for wealth, power, fame or enjoyment, the yogi has one craving and that is to adore the Lord. Freedom from craving enables one to ward off great temptations. Craving muddies the stream of tranquillity. It makes men base and vile and cripples them. He who obeys the commandment *Thou shalt not steal,* becomes a trusted repository of all treasures.

Brahmacharya. According to the dictionary brahmacharya means the life of celibacy, religious study and self-restraint. It is thought that the loss of semen leads to death and its retention to life. By the preservation of semen the yogi's body develops a sweet smell. So long as it is retained, there is no fear of death. Hence the injunction that it should be preserved by concentrated effort of the mind. The concept of brahmacharya is not one of negation, forced austerity and prohibition. According to Śankarāchārya, a brahmachārī (one who observes brahmacharya) is a man who is engrossed in the study of the sacred Vedic lore, constantly moves in Brahman and knows that all exists in Brahman. In other words, one who sees divinity in all is a brahmachārī. Patañjali, however, lays stress on continence of the body, speech and mind. This does not mean that the philosophy of Yoga is meant only for celibates. Brahmacharya has little to do with whether one is a bachelor or married and living the life of a householder. One has to develop the higher aspects of Brahmacharya in one's daily living. It is not necessary for one's salvation to stay unmarried and without a house. On the contrary, all the smṛtīs (codes of law) recommend marriage. Without experiencing human love and happiness, it is not possible to know divine love. Almost all the yogis and sages of old in India were married men with families of their own. They did not shirk their social or moral responsibilities. Marriage and parenthood are no bar to the knowledge of divine love, happiness and union with the Supreme Soul.

Dealing with the position of an aspirant who is a householder, the *Śiva Saṁhitā* says: Let him practise free from the company of men in a retired place. For the sake of appearances, he should remain in society, but not have his heart in it. He should not renounce the duties of his profession, caste or rank; but let him perform these as an instrument of the Lord, without any thought of the results. He succeeds by following wisely the method of Yoga; there is no doubt of it. Remaining in the midst of the family, always doing the duties of the householder, he who is free from merits and demerits and has restrained his senses, attains salvation. The householder practising Yoga is not touched by virtue or vice; if to protect mankind he commits any sin, he is not polluted by it. (Chapter V, verses 234–8.)

When one is established in brahmacharya, one develops a fund of vitality and energy, a courageous mind and a powerful intellect so that one can fight any type of injustice. The brahmachārī will use the forces he generates wisely: he will utilise the physical ones for doing the work of the Lord, the mental for the spread of culture and the intellectual for the growth of spiritual life. Brahmacharya is the battery that sparks the torch of wisdom.

Aparigraha. Parigraha means hoarding or collecting. To be free from hoarding is aparigraha. It is thus but another facet of asteya (non-stealing). Just as one should not take things one does not really need, so one should not hoard or collect things one does not require immediately. Neither should one take anything without working for it or as a favour from another, for this indicates poverty of spirit. The yogi feels that the collection or hoarding of things implies a lack of faith in God and in himself to provide for his future. He keeps faith by keeping before him the image of the moon. During the dark half of the month, the moon rises late when most men are asleep and so do not appreciate its beauty. Its splendour wanes but it does not stray from its path and is indifferent to man's lack of appreciation. It has faith that it will be full again when it faces the Sun and then men will eagerly await its glorious rising.

By the observance of aparigraha, the yogi makes his life as simple as possible and trains his mind not to feel the loss or the lack of anything. Then everything he really needs will come to him by itself at the proper time. The life of an ordinary man is filled with an unending series of disturbances and frustrations and with his reactions to them. Thus there is hardly any possibility of keeping the mind in a state of equilibrium. The sādhaka has developed the capacity to remain satisfied with whatever happens to him. Thus he obtains the peace which takes him beyond the realms of illusion and misery with which our world is saturated. He recalls the promise given by Śri Krishna to Arjuna in the ninth chapter of the *Bhagavad Gītā*: 'To those who worship Me alone with single-minded devotion, who are in harmony with Me every moment, I bring full security. I shall supply all their wants and shall protect them for ever.'

Niyama

Niyama are the rules of conduct that apply to individual discipline, while yama are universal in their application. The five niyama listed by Patañjali are: śaucha (purity), santoṣa (contentment), tapas (ardour or austerity), svādhyāya (study of the Self) and Iśvara praṇidhāna (dedication to the Lord).

Śaucha. Purity of body is essential for well-being. While good habits like bathing purify the body externally, āsana and prāṇāyāma cleanse it internally. The practice of āsanas tones the entire body and removes the toxins and impurities caused by over-indulgence. Prāṇāyāma cleanses and aerates the lungs, oxygenates the blood and purifies the nerves. But more important than the physical cleansing of the body is the cleansing of the mind of its disturbing emotions like hatred, passion, anger, lust, greed, delusion and pride. Still more important is the cleansing of the intellect (buddhi) of impure thoughts. The impurities of the mind are washed off in the waters of bhakti (adoration). The impurities of the intellect or reason are burned off in the fire of svādhyāya (study of the Self). This internal cleansing gives radiance and joy. It brings benevolence (saumanasya) and banishes mental pain, dejection, sorrow and despair (daurmanasya). When one is benevolent, one sees the virtues in others and not merely their faults. The respect which one shows for another's virtues, makes him self-respecting as well and helps him to fight his own sorrows and difficulties. When the mind is lucid, it is easy to make it one-pointed (ekāgra). With concentration, one obtains mastery over the senses (indriya-jaya). Then one is ready to enter the temple of his own body and see his real self in the mirror of his mind.

Besides purity of body, thought and word, pure food is also necessary. Apart from cleanliness in the preparation of food it is also necessary to observe purity in the means by which one procures it.

Food, the supporting yet consuming substance of all life, is regarded as a phase of Brahman. It should be eaten with the feeling that with each morsel one can gain strength to serve the Lord. Then food becomes pure. Whether or not to be a vegetarian is a purely personal matter as each person is influenced by the tradition and habits of the country in which he was born and bred. But, in course of time, the practitioner of yoga has to adopt a vegetarian diet, in order to attain one-pointed attention and spiritual evolution.

Food should be taken to promote health, strength, energy and life. It should be simple, nourishing, juicy and soothing. Avoid foods which are sour, bitter, pungent, burning, stale, tasteless, heavy and unclean.

Character is moulded by the type of food we take and by how we eat it. Men are the only creatures that eat when not hungry and generally live to eat rather than eat to live. If we eat for flavours of the tongue, we over-eat and so suffer from digestive disorders which throw our systems out of gear. The yogi believes in harmony, so he eats for the sake of sustenance only. He does not eat too much or too little. He looks upon his body as the rest-house of his spirit and guards himself against over-indulgence.

Besides food, the place is also important for spiritual practices. It is difficult to practise in a distant country (away from home), in a forest, in a crowded city, or where it is noisy. One should choose a place where food is easily procurable, a place which is free from insects, protected from the elements and with pleasing surroundings. The banks of a lake or river or the sea-shore are ideal. Such quiet ideal places are hard to find in modern times; but one can at least make a corner in one's room available for practice and keep it clean, airy, dry and pest-free.

Santoṣa. Santoṣa or contentment has to be cultivated. A mind that is not content cannot concentrate. The yogi feels the lack of nothing and so he is naturally content. Contentment gives bliss unsurpassed to the yogi. A contented man is complete for he has known the love of the Lord and has done his duty. He is blessed for he has known truth and joy.

Contentment and tranquillity are states of mind. Differences arise among men because of race, creed, wealth and learning. Differences create discord and there arise conscious or unconscious conflicts which distract and perplex one. Then the mind cannot become one-pointed (ekāgra) and is robbed of its peace. There is contentment and tranquillity when the flame of the spirit does not waver in the wind of desire. The sādhaka does not seek the empty peace of the dead, but the peace of one whose reason is firmly established in God.

Tapas. Tapas is derived from the root 'tap' meaning to blaze, burn, shine, suffer pain or consume by heat. It therefore means a burning effort under all circumstances to achieve a definite goal in life. It involves purification, self-discipline and austerity. The whole science of character building may be regarded as a practice of tapas.

Tapas is the conscious effort to achieve ultimate union with the Divine and to burn up all desires which stand in the way of this goal. A worthy aim makes life illumined, pure and divine. Without such an aim, action and prayer have no value. Life without tapas, is like a heart without love. Without tapas, the mind cannot reach up to the Lord.

Tapas is of three types. It may relate to the body (kāyika), to speech (vāchika) or to mind (mānasika). Continence (brahmacharya) and non-violence (ahimsā) are tapas of the body. Using words which do not offend, reciting the glory of God, speaking the truth without regard for the consequences to oneself and not speaking ill of others are tapas of speech. Developing a mental attitude whereby one remains tranquil and balanced in joy and sorrow and retains self-control are tapas of the mind.

It is tapas when one works without any selfish motive or hope of reward and with an unshakable faith that not even a blade of grass can move without His will.

By tapas the yogi develops strength in body, mind and character. He gains courage and wisdom, integrity, straightforwardness and simplicity.

Svādhyāya. Sva means self and adhyāya means study or education. Education is the drawing out of the best that is within a person. Svādhyāya, therefore, is the education of the self.

Svādhyāya is different from mere instruction like attending a lecture where the lecturer parades his own learning before the ignorance of his audience. When people meet for svādhyāya, the speaker and listener are of one mind and have mutual love and respect. There is no sermonising and one heart speaks to another. The ennobling thoughts that arise from svādhyāya are, so to speak, taken into one's bloodstream so that they become a part of one's life and being.

The person practising svādhyāya reads his own book of

life, at the same time that he writes and revises it. There is a change in his outlook on life. He starts to realise that all creation is meant for bhakti (adoration) rather than for bhoga (enjoyment), that all creation is divine, that there is divinity within himself and that the energy which moves him is the same that moves the entire universe.

According to Śri Vinobā Bhāve (the leader of the Bhoodan movement), svādhyāya is the study of one subject which is the basis or root of all other subjects or actions, upon which the others rest, but which itself does not rest upon anything.

To make life healthy, happy and peaceful, it is essential to study regularly divine literature in a pure place. This study of the sacred books of the world will enable the sādhaka to concentrate upon and solve the difficult problems of life when they arise. It will put an end to ignorance and bring knowledge. Ignorance has no beginning, but it has an end. There is a beginning but no end to knowledge. By svādhyāya the sādhaka understands the nature of his soul and gains communion with the divine. The sacred books of the world are for all to read. They are not meant for the members of one particular faith alone. As bees savour the nectar in various flowers, so the sādhaka absorbs things in other faiths which will enable him to appreciate his own faith better.

Philology is not a language but the science of languages, the study of which will enable the student to learn his own language better. Similarly, Yoga is not a religion by itself. It is the science of religions, the study of which will enable a sādhaka the better to appreciate his own faith.

Īśvara praṇidhāna. Dedication to the Lord of one's actions and will is Īśvara praṇidhāna. He who has faith in God does not despair. He has illumination (tejas). He who knows that all creation belongs to the Lord will not be puffed up with pride or drunk with power. He will not stoop for selfish purposes; his head will bow only in worship. When the waters of bhakti (adoration) are made to flow through the turbines of the mind, the result is mental power and spiritual illumination. While mere physical strength without bhakti is lethal, mere adoration without strength of character is like an opiate. Addiction to pleasures destroys both power and glory. From the gratification of the senses as they run after pleasures arise moha (attachment) and lobha (greed) for their repetition. If the senses are not gratified, then, there is śoka (sorrow). They have to be curbed with knowledge and forbearance; but to control the mind is more difficult. After one has exhausted one's own resources and still not succeeded, one turns to the Lord for help for He is the source of all power. It is at this stage that bhakti begins. In bhakti, the mind, the intellect and the will are surrendered to the Lord and the sādhaka prays: 'I do not know what is good for me. Thy will be done.' Others pray to have their own desires gratified or accomplished. In bhakti or true love there is no place for 'I' and 'mine'. When the feeling of 'I' and 'mine' disappears, the individual soul has reached full growth.

When the mind has been emptied of desires of personal gratification, it should be filled with thoughts of the Lord. In a mind filled with thoughts of personal gratification, there is danger of the senses dragging the mind after the objects of desire. Attempts to practise bhakti without emptying the mind of desires is like building a fire with wet fuel. It makes a lot of smoke and brings tears to the eyes of the person who builds it and of those around him. A mind with desires does not ignite and glow, nor does it generate light and warmth when touched with the fire of knowledge.

The name of the Lord is like the Sun, dispelling all darkness. The moon is full when it faces the sun. The individual soul experiences fullness (pūrṇatā) when it faces the Lord. If the shadow of the earth comes between the full moon and the sun there is an eclipse. If the feeling of 'I' and 'mine' casts its shadow upon the experience of fullness, all efforts of the sādhaka to gain peace are futile.

Actions mirror a man's personality better than his words. The yogi has learnt the art of dedicating all his actions to the Lord and so they reflect the divinity within him.

Āsana

The third limb of yoga is āsana or posture. Āsana brings steadiness, health and lightness of limb. A steady and pleasant posture produces mental equilibrium and prevents fickleness of mind. Āsanas are not merely gymnastic exercises; they are postures. To perform them one needs a clean airy place, a blanket and determination, while for other systems of physical training one needs large playing fields and costly equipment. Āsanas can be done alone, as the limbs of the body provide the necessary weights and counter-weights. By practising them one develops agility, balance, endurance and great vitality.

Āsanas have been evolved over the centuries so as to exercise every muscle, nerve and gland in the body. They secure a fine physique, which is strong and elastic without being muscle-bound and they keep the body free from disease. They reduce fatigue and soothe the nerves. But their real importance lies in the way they train and discipline the mind.

Many actors, acrobats, athletes, dancers, musicians and sportsmen also possess superb physiques and have great control over the body, but they lack control over the mind, the intellect and the Self. Hence they are in disharmony with themselves and one rarely comes across a balanced personality among them. They often put the body above all else. Though the yogi does not underrate his body, he does not think merely of its perfection but of his senses, mind, intellect and soul.

The yogi conquers the body by the practice of āsanas and makes it a fit vehicle for the spirit. He knows that it is a necessary vehicle for the spirit. A soul without a body is like a bird deprived of its power to fly.

The yogi does not fear death, for time must take its toll of all flesh. He knows that the body is constantly changing and is affected by childhood, youth and old age. Birth and death are natural phenomena but the soul is not subject to birth and death. As a man casting off worn-out garments takes on new ones, so the dweller within the body casting aside worn-out bodies enters into others that are new.

The yogi believes that his body has been given to him by the Lord not for enjoyment alone, but also for the service of his fellow men during every wakeful moment of his life. He does not consider it his property. He knows that the Lord who has given him his body will one day take it away.

By performing āsanas, the sādhaka first gains health, which is not mere existence. It is not a commodity which can be purchased with money. It is an asset to be gained by sheer hard work. It is a state of complete equilibrium of body, mind and spirit. Forgetfulness of physical and mental consciousness is health. The yogi frees himself from physical disabilities and mental distractions by practising āsanas. He surrenders his actions and their fruits to the Lord in the service of the world.

The yogi realises that his life and all its activities are part of the divine action in nature, manifesting and operating in the form of man. In the beating of his pulse and the rhythm of his respiration, he recognises the flow of the seasons and the throbbing of universal life. His body is a temple which houses the Divine Spark. He feels that to neglect or to deny the needs of the body and to think of it as something not divine, is to neglect and deny the universal life of which it is a part. The needs of the body are the needs of the divine spirit which lives through the body. The yogi does not look heaven-ward to find God for he knows that He is within, being known as the Antarātmā (the Inner Self). He feels the kingdom of God within and without and finds that heaven lies in himself.

Where does the body end and the mind begin? Where does the mind end and the spirit begin? They cannot be divided as they are inter-related and but different aspects of the same all-pervading divine consciousness.

The yogi never neglects or mortifies the body or the mind, but cherishes both. To him the body is not an impediment to his spiritual liberation nor is it the cause of its fall, but is an instrument of attainment. He seeks a body strong as a thunderbolt, healthy and free from suffering so as to dedicate it in the service of the Lord for which it is intended. As pointed out in the *Muṇḍakopaniṣad* the Self cannot be attained by one without strength, nor through heedlessness, nor without an aim. Just as an unbaked earthen pot dissolves in water the body soon decays. So bake it hard in the fire of yogic discipline in order to strengthen and purify it.

The names of the āsanas are significant and illustrate the principle of evolution. Some are named after vegetation like the tree (vṛkṣa) and the lotus (padma); some after insects like the locust (śalabha) and the scorpion (vṛśchika); some after aquatic animals and amphibians like the fish (matsya), the tortoise (kūrma), the frog (bheka or maṇḍūka) or the crocodile (nakra). There are āsanas called after birds like the cock (kukkuṭa), the heron (baka), the peacock (mayūra) and the swan (haṁsa). They are also named after quadrupeds like the dog (śvāna), the horse (vātāyana), the camel (uṣṭra) and the lion (siṁha). Creatures that crawl like the serpent (bhujaṅga) are not forgotten, nor is the human embryonic state (garbha-pinda) overlooked. Āsanas are named after legendary heroes like Vīrabhadra and Hanumān, son of the Wind. Sages like Bharadvāja, Kapila, Vasiṣṭha and Viśvāmitra are remembered by having āsanas named after them. Some āsanas are also called after gods of the Hindu pantheon and some recall the Avatārās, or incarnations of Divine Power. Whilst performing āsanas the yogi's body assumes many forms resembling a variety of creatures. His mind is trained not to despise any creature, for he knows that throughout the whole gamut of creation, from the lowliest insect to the most perfect sage, there breathes the same Universal Spirit, which assumes innumerable forms. He knows that the highest form is that of the Formless. He finds unity in universality. True āsana is that in which the thought of Brahman flows effortlessly and incessantly through the mind of the sādhaka.

Dualities like gain and loss, victory and defeat, fame and shame, body and mind, mind and soul vanish through mastery of the āsanas, and the sādhaka then passes on to prāṇāyāma, the fourth stage in the path of yoga. In prāṇāyāma practices the nostrils, nasal passages and membranes, the windpipe, the lungs and the diaphragm are the only parts of the body which are actively involved. These alone feel the full impact of the force of prāṇa, the breath of life. Therefore, do not seek to master prāṇāyāma in a hurry, as you are playing with life itself. By its improper practice respiratory diseases will arise and the nervous system will be shattered. By its proper practice one is freed from most diseases. Never attempt to practise prāṇāyāma alone by yourself. For it is essential to have the personal supervision of a Guru who knows the physical limitations of his pupil.

Prāṇāyāma

Just as the word yoga is one of wide import, so also is prāṇa. Prāṇa means breath, respiration, life, vitality, wind, energy or strength. It also connotes the soul as opposed to the body. The word is generally used in the plural to indicate vital breaths. Āyāma means length, expansion, stretching or restraint. Prāṇāyāma thus connotes extension of breath and its control. This control is over all the functions of breathing, namely, (1) inhalation or inspiration, which is termed pūraka (filling up); (2) exhalation or expiration, which is called rechaka (emptying the lungs), and (3) retention or holding the breath, a state where there is no inhalation or exhalation, which is termed kumbhaka. In Haṭha Yoga texts kumbhaka is also used in a loose generic sense to include all the three respiratory processes of inhalation, exhalation and retention.

A kumbha is a pitcher, water pot, jar or chalice. A water pot may be emptied of all air and filled completely with water, or it may be emptied of all water and filled completely with air. Similarly, there are two states of kumbhaka namely (1) when breathing is suspended after full inhalation (the lungs being completely filled with life-giving air), and (2) when breathing is suspended after full exhalation (the lungs being emptied of all noxious air). The first of these states, where breath is held after a full inhalation, but before exhalation begins, is known as antara kumbhaka. The second, where breath is held after a full exhalation, but before inhalation begins is known as bāhya kumbhaka. Antara means inner or interior, while bāhya means outer or exterior. Thus, kumbhaka is the interval or intermediate time between full inhalation and exhalation (antara kumbhaka) or between full exhalation and inhalation (bāhya kumbhaka). In both these types breathing is suspended and restrained.

Prāṇāyāma is thus the science of breath. It is the hub round which the wheel of life revolves. 'As lions, elephants and tigers are tamed very slowly and cautiously, so should prāṇa be brought under control very slowly in gradation measured according to one's capacity and physical limitations. Otherwise it will kill the practitioner,' warns the *Haṭha Yoga Pradīpikā* (chapter II, verse 16).

The yogi's life is not measured by the number of his days but by the number of his breaths. Therefore, he follows the proper rhythmic patterns of slow deep breathing. These rhythmic patterns strengthen the respiratory system, soothe the nervous system and reduce craving. As desires and cravings diminish, the mind is set free and becomes a fit vehicle for concentration. By improper practice of prāṇāyāma the pupil introduces several disorders into his system like hiccough, wind, asthma, cough, catarrh, pains in the head, eyes and ears and nervous irritation. It takes a long time to learn slow, deep, steady and proper inhalations and exhalations. Master this before attempting kumbhaka.

As a fire blazes brightly when the covering of ash over it is scattered by the wind, the divine fire within the body shines in all its majesty when the ashes of desire are scattered by the practice of prāṇāyāma.

'The emptying the mind of the whole of its illusion is the true rechaka (exhalation). The realisation that "I am Ātmā (spirit)" is the true pūraka (inhalation). And the steady sustenance of the mind on this conviction is the true kumbhaka (retention). This is true prāṇāyāma,' says Śankarāchārya.

Every living creature unconsciously breathes the prayer 'So'ham' (Saḥ=He:Aham=I–He, the Immortal Spirit, am I) with each inward breath. So also with each outgoing breath each creature prays 'Haṁsaḥ' (I am He). This ajapa-mantra (unconscious repetitive prayer) goes on for ever within each living creature throughout life. The yogi fully realises the significance of this ajapa-mantra and so is released from all the fetters that bind his soul. He offers up the very breath of his being to the Lord as a sacrifice and receives the breath of life from the Lord as his blessing.

Prāṇa in the body of the individual (jīvātmā) is part of the cosmic breath of the Universal Spirit (Paramātmā). An attempt is made to harmonise the individual breath (piṇḍa-prāṇa) with the cosmic breath (Brahmāṇḍa-prāṇa) through the practice of prāṇāyāma.

It has been said by Kariba Ekken, a seventeenth-century mystic: 'If you would foster a calm spirit, first regulate your breathing; for when that is under control, the heart will be at peace; but when breathing is spasmodic, then it will be troubled. Therefore, before attempting anything, first regulate your breathing on which your temper will be softened, your spirit calmed.'

The chitta (mind, reason and ego) is like a chariot yoked to a team of powerful horses. One of them is prāṇa (breath), the other is vāsanā (desire). The chariot moves in the direction of the more powerful animal. If breath prevails, the desires are controlled, the senses are held in check and the mind is stilled. If desire prevails, breath is in disarray and the mind is agitated and troubled. Therefore, the yogi masters the science of breath and by the regulation and control of breath, he controls the mind and stills its constant movement. In the practice of prāṇāyāma the eyes are kept shut to prevent the mind from wandering. 'When the prāṇa and the manas (mind) have been absorbed, an undefinable joy ensues.' (*Haṭha Yoga Pradīpikā*, chapter IV, verse 30.)

Emotional excitement affects the rate of breathing; equally, deliberate regulation of breathing checks emotional excitement. As the very object of Yoga is to control and still the mind, the yogi first learns prāṇāyāma to master the breath. This will enable him to control the senses and so reach the stage of pratyāhāra. Only then will the mind be ready for concentration (dhyāna).

The mind is said to be twofold – pure and impure. It is pure when it is completely free from desires and impure when it is in union with desires. By making the mind motionless and freeing it from sloth and distractions, one reaches the state of mindlessness (amanaska), which is the supreme state of samādhi. This state of mindlessness is not lunacy or idiocy but the conscious state of the mind when it is free from thoughts and desires. There is a vital difference between an idiot or a lunatic on the one hand, and a yogi striving to achieve a state of mindlessness on the other. The former is careless; the latter attempts to be carefree. It is the oneness of the breath and mind and so also of the senses and the abandonment of all conditions of existence and thought that is designated Yoga.

Prāṇa Vāyu. One of the most subtle forms of energy is air. This vital energy which also pervades the human body is classified in five main categories in the Haṭha Yoga texts according to the various functions performed by the energy. These are termed vāyu (wind) and the five main divisions are: prāṇa (here the generic term is used to designate the particular), which moves in the region of the heart and controls respiration; apāna, which moves in the sphere of the lower abdomen and controls the function of eliminating urine and faeces; samāna, which stokes the gastric fires to aid digestion; udāna, which dwells in the thoracic cavity and controls the intake of air and food; and vyāna, which pervades the entire body and distributes the energy derived from food and breath. There are also five subsidiary vāyūs. These are: nāga, which relieves abdominal pressure by belching; kūrma, which controls the movements of the eyelids to prevent foreign matter or too bright a light entering the eyes; kṛkara, which prevents substances passing up the nasal passages and down the throat by making one sneeze or cough; devadatta, which provides for the intake of extra oxygen in a tired body by causing a yawn, and lastly dhanaṁjaya, which remains in the body even after death and sometimes bloats up a corpse.

Pratyāhāra

If a man's reason succumbs to the pull of his senses he is lost. On the other hand, if there is rhythmic control of breath, the senses instead of running after external objects of desire turn inwards, and man is set free from their tyranny. This is the fifth stage of Yoga, namely, pratyāhāra, where the senses are brought under control.

When this stage is reached, the sādhaka goes through a searching self-examination. To overcome the deadly but attractive spell of sensual objects, he needs the insulation of adoration (bhakti) by recalling to his mind the Creator who made the objects of his desire. He also needs the lamp of knowledge of his divine heritage. The mind, in truth, is for mankind the cause of bondage and liberation; it brings bondage if it is bound to the objects of desire and liberation when it is free from objects. There is bondage when the mind craves, grieves or is unhappy over something. The mind becomes pure when all desires and fears are annihilated. Both the good and the pleasant present themselves to men and prompt them to action. The yogi prefers the good to the pleasant. Others driven by their desires, prefer the pleasant to the good and miss the very purpose of life. The yogi feels joy in what he is. He knows how to stop and, therefore, lives in peace. At first he prefers that which is bitter as poison, but he perseveres in his practice knowing well that in the end it will become as sweet as nectar. Others hankering for the union of their senses with the objects of their desires, prefer that which at first seems sweet as nectar, but do not know that in the end it will be as bitter as poison.

The yogi knows that the path towards satisfaction of the senses by sensual desires is broad, but that it leads to destruction and that there are many who follow it. The path of Yoga is like the sharp edge of a razor, narrow and difficult to tread, and there are few who find it. The yogi knows that the paths of ruin or of salvation lie within himself.

According to Hindu philosophy, consciousness manifests in three different qualities. For man, his life and his consciousness, together with the entire cosmos are the emanations of one and the same prakṛti (cosmic matter or substance) – emanations that differ in designation through the predominance of one of the guṇās. The guṇās (qualities or attributes) are:

1 Sattva (the illuminating, pure or good quality), which leads to clarity and mental serenity.
2 Rajas (the quality of mobility or activity), which makes a person active and energetic, tense and wilful, and

3 Tamas (the dark and restraining quality), which obstructs and counteracts the tendency of rajas to work and of sattva to reveal.

Tamas is a quality of delusion, obscurity, inertia and ignorance. A person in whom it predominates is inert and plunged in a state of torpor. The quality of sattva leads towards the divine and tamas towards the demonic, while in between these two stands rajas.

The faith held, the food consumed, the sacrifices performed, the austerities undergone and the gifts given by each individual vary in accordance with his predominating guṇa.

He that is born with tendencies towards the divine is fearless and pure. He is generous and self-controlled. He pursues the study of the Self. He is non-violent, truthful and free from anger. He renounces the fruits of his labour, working only for the sake of work. He has a tranquil mind, with malice towards none and charity towards all, for he is free from craving. He is gentle, modest and steady. He is illumined, clement and resolute, being free from perfidy and pride.

A man in whom rajō-guṇa predominates has inner thirst. As he is passionate and covetous, he hurts others. Being full of lust and hatred, envy and deceit, his desires are insatiable. He is unsteady, fickle and easily distracted as well as ambitious and acquisitive. He seeks the patronage of friends and has family pride. He shrinks from unpleasant things and clings to pleasant ones. His speech is sour and his stomach greedy.

He that is born with demonic tendencies is deceitful, insolent and conceited. He is full of wrath, cruelty and ignorance. In such people there is neither purity, nor right conduct, nor truth. They gratify their passions. Bewildered by numerous desires, caught in the web of delusion, these addicts of sensual pleasures fall into hell.

The working of the mind of persons with different predominating gunās may be illustrated by their different ways of approach towards a universal commandment like 'Thou shalt not covet.' A man in whom tamō-guṇa predominates might interpret it thus: 'others should not covet what is mine, no matter how I obtained it. If they do, I shall destroy them.' The rajō-guṇa type is a calculating self-interested person who would construe the commandment as meaning: 'I will not covet others' goods lest they covet mine.' He will follow the letter of the law as a matter of policy, but not the true spirit of the law as a matter of principle. A person of sattvika temperament will follow both the letter and the spirit of the precept as a matter of principle and not of policy, as a matter of eternal value. He will be righteous for the sake of righteousness alone, and not because there is a human law imposing punishment to keep him honest.

The yogi who is also human is affected by these three guṇās. By his constant and disciplined study (abhyāsa) of himself and of the objects which his senses tend to pursue, he learns which thoughts, words and actions are prompted by tamas and which by rajas. With unceasing effort he weeds out and eradicates such thoughts and he works to achieve a sattvika frame of mind. When the sattva-guṇa alone remains, the human soul has advanced a long way towards the ultimate goal.

Like unto the pull of gravity is the pull of the guṇās. As intensive research and rigorous discipline are needed to experience the wonder of weightlessness in space, so also a searching self-examination and the discipline furnished by Yoga is needed by a sādhaka to experience union with the Creator of space when he is freed from the pull of the guṇās.

Once the sādhaka has experienced the fullness of creation or of the Creator, his thirst (tṛṣṇā) for objects of sense vanishes and he looks at them ever after with dispassion (vairāgya). He experiences no disquiet in heat or cold, in pain or pleasure, in honour or dishonour and in virtue or vice. He treats the two imposters – triumph and disaster – with equanimity. He has emancipated himself from these pairs of opposites. He has passed beyond the pull of the guṇās and has become a guṇātīta (one who has transcended the guṇās). He is then free from birth and death, from pain and sorrow and becomes immortal. He has no self-identity as he lives experiencing the fullness of the Universal Soul. Such a man, scorning nothing, leads all things to the path of perfection.

Dhāranā

When the body has been tempered by āsanas, when the mind has been refined by the fire of prāṇāyāma and when the senses have been brought under control by pratyāhāra, the sādhaka reaches the sixth stage called dhāraṇā. Here he is concentrated wholly on a single point or on a task in which he is completely engrossed. The mind has to be stilled in order to achieve this state of complete absorption.

The mind is an instrument which classifies, judges and co-ordinates the impressions from the outside world and those that arise within oneself.

Mind is the product of thoughts which are difficult to restrain for they are subtle and fickle. A thought which is well guarded by a controlled mind brings happiness. To get the best out of an instrument, one must know how it works. The mind is the instrument for thinking and it is therefore necessary to consider how it functions. Mental states are classified in five groups. The first of these is the kṣipta state, where the mental forces are scattered, being in disarray and in a state of neglect. Here the mind hankers after objects, the ragō-guṇa being dominant. The second is the vikṣipta state, where the mind is agitated and distracted. Here there is a capacity to enjoy the fruits of one's efforts, but the desires are not marshalled and controlled. Then in the mūḍha state the mind is foolish, dull and stupid. It is confounded and at a loss to know what it wants and here the tamō-guṇa predominates. The fourth state of the mind is the ekāgra (eka=one; agra= foremost) state, where the mind is closely attentive and the mental faculties are concentrated on a single object or focussed on one point only, with the sattva-guṇa prevailing. The ekāgra person has superior intellectual powers and knows exactly what he wants, so he uses all his powers to achieve his purpose. At times the ruthless pursuit of the desired object, irrespective of the cost to others, can create great misery, and it often happens that even if the desired object is achieved it leaves behind a bitter taste.

Arjuna, the mighty bowman of the epic Mahābhārata,

provides us with an example of what is meant by dhāraṇā. Once Drona, the preceptor of the royal princes, organised an archery contest to test their proficiency. They were called upon one by one to describe the target, which was pointed out to them. It was a nesting bird. Some princes described the grove of trees, others the particular tree or the bough on which the nest stood. When Arjuna's turn came, he described first the bird. Then he saw only its head, and lastly he could see nothing but the shining eye of the bird, which was the centre of the target chosen by Droṇa.

There is danger, however, of an ekāgra person becoming supremely egotistical. Where the senses start roaming unchecked, the mind follows suit. They cloud a man's judgement and set him adrift like a battered ship on a storm-tossed sea. A ship needs ballast to keep her on an even keel and the helmsman needs a star to steer her by. The ekāgra person needs bhakti (adoration of the Lord) and concentration on divinity to keep his mental equilibrium so that he goes on always in the right direction. He will not know happiness until the sense of 'I' and 'mine' disappears.

The last mental state is that of niruddha, where the mind (manas), intellect (buddhi) and ego (ahaṁkāra) are all restrained and all these faculties are offered to the Lord for His use and in His service. Here there is no feeling of 'I' and 'mine'. As a lens becomes more luminous when great light is thrown upon it and seems to be all light and undistinguishable from it, so also the sādhaka who has given up his mind, intellect and ego to the Lord, becomes one with Him, for the sādhaka thinks of nothing but Him, who is the creator of thought.

Without ekāgratā or concentration one can master nothing. Without concentration on Divinity, which shapes and controls the universe, one cannot unlock the divinity within oneself or become a universal man. To achieve this concentration, what is recommended is eka-tattva-abhyāsa or study of the single element that pervades all, the inmost Self of all beings, who converts His one form into many. The sādhaka, therefore, concentrates upon AUM, which is His symbol, to achieve ekāgratā.

Aum: According to Śri Vinobā Bhāve, the Latin word Omne and the Sanskrit word Aum are both derived from the same root meaning all and both words convey the concepts of omniscience, omnipresence and omnipotence. Another word for Aum is praṇava, which is derived from the root nu meaning to praise, to which is added the prefix pra denoting superiority. The word, therefore, means the best praise or the best prayer.

The symbol AUM is composed of three syllables, namely the letters A, U, M, and when written has a crescent and dot on its top. A few instances of the various interpretations given to it may be mentioned here to convey its meaning.

The letter A symbolises the conscious or waking state (jāgrata-avasthā), the letter U the dream state (svapna-avasthā) and the letter M the dreamless sleep state (suṣupta-avasthā) of the mind and spirit. The entire symbol, together with the crescent and the dot, stands for the fourth state (turīya-avasthā), which combines all these states and transcends them. This is the state of samādhi.

The letters A, U and M symbolise respectively speech (vak), the mind (manas) and the breath of life (prāṇa), while the entire symbol stands for the living spirit, which is but a portion of the divine spirit.

The three letters also represent the dimensions of length, breadth and depth, while the entire symbol represents Divinity, which is beyond the limitations of shape and form.

The three letters A, U and M symbolise the absence of desire, fear and anger, while the whole symbol stands for the perfect man (a sthita-prajñā), one whose wisdom is firmly established in the divine.

They represent the three genders, masculine, feminine and neuter, while the entire symbol represents all creation together with the Creator.

They stand for the three guṇās or qualities of sattva, rajas and tamas, while the whole symbol represents a guṇātīta, one who has transcended and gone beyond the pull of the guṇās.

The letters correspond to the three tenses – past, present and future – while the entire symbol stands for the Creator, who transcends the limitations of time.

They also stand for the teaching imparted by the mother, the father and the Guru respectively. The entire symbol represents Brahma Vidyā, the knowledge of the Self, the teaching which is imperishable.

The A, U and M depict the three stages of yogic discipline, namely, āsana, prāṇāyāma and pratyāhāra. The entire symbol represents samādhi, the goal for which the three stages are the steps.

They represent the triad of Divinity, namely, Brahmā – the creator, Viṣṇu – the Maintainer, and Śiva – the Destroyer of the universe. The whole symbol is said to represent Brahman from which the universe emanates, has its growth and fruition and into which it merges in the end. It does not grow or change. Many change and pass, but Brahman is the One that ever remains unchanged.

The letters A, U and M also stand for the mantra 'Tat Twam Asi' ('That Thou Art'), the realisation of man's divinity within himself. The entire symbol stands for this realisation, which liberates the human spirit from the confines of his body, mind, intellect and ego.

After realising the importance of AUM, the yogi focusses his attention on his beloved Deity adding AUM to the name of the Lord. The word AUM being too vast and too abstract, he unifies his senses, will, intellect, mind and reason by focussing on the name of the Lord and adding the word AUM with one pointed devotion and so experiences the feeling and meaning of the mantra.

The yogi recalls the verses of the *Muṇḍakopaniṣad*: 'Taking as a bow the great weapon of the Upaniṣad, one should put upon it an arrow sharpened by meditation. Stretching it with a thought directed to the essence of That, penetrate the Imperishable as the mark, my friend. The mystic syllable AUM is the bow. The arrow is the Self (Ātmā). Brahman is the target. By the undistracted man is It penetrated. One should come to be in It, as the arrow in the mark.'

Dhyāna

As water takes the shape of its container, the mind when it contemplates an object is transformed into the shape of that object. The mind which thinks of the all-pervading divinity which it worships, is ultimately through long-continued devotion transformed into the likeness of that divinity.

When oil is poured from one vessel to another, one can observe the steady constant flow. When the flow of concentration is uninterrupted, the state that arises is dhyāna (meditation). As the filament in an electric bulb glows and illumines when there is a regular uninterrupted current of electricity, the yogi's mind will be illumined by dhyāna. His body, breath, senses, mind, reason and ego are all integrated in the object of his contemplation – the Universal Spirit. He remains in a state of consciousness which has no qualification whatsoever. There is no other feeling except a state of SUPREME BLISS. Like a streak of lightning the yogi sees LIGHT that shines beyond the earth and the heavens. He sees the light that shines in his own heart. He becomes a light unto himself and others.

The signs of progress on the path of Yoga are health, a sense of physical lightness, steadiness, clearness of countenance and a beautiful voice, sweetness of odour of the body and freedom from craving. He has a balanced, serene and a tranquil mind. He is the very symbol of humility. He dedicates all his actions to the Lord and taking refuge in Him, frees himself from the bondage of karma (action) and becomes a Jīvana Mukta (a Liberated Soul).

'What becomes of him who strives and fails to reach the end of Yoga, who has faith, but whose mind wanders away from Yoga?' To this query of Arjuna, the Lord Śri Krishna replied:

'No evil can befall a righteous man. He dwells long years in the heaven of those who did good, and then he is reborn in the house of the pure and the great. He may even be born in a family of illumined yogis; but to be born in such a family is most difficult in this world. He will regain the wisdom attained in his former life and strives ever for perfection. Because of his former study, practice and struggle which drive him ever onwards, the yogi ever strives with a soul cleansed of sin, attains perfection through many lives and reaches the supreme goal. The yogi goes beyond those who only follow the path of austerity, knowledge or service. Therefore, Arjuna, be thou a yogi. The greatest of all yogis is he who adores Me with faith and whose heart abides in Me.' (*Bhagavad Gītā*, chapter VI, verses 38 to 47.)

Samādhi

Samādhi is the end of the sādhaka's quest. At the peak of his meditation, he passes into the state of samādhi, where his body and senses are at rest as if he is asleep, his faculties of mind and reason are alert as if he is awake, yet he has gone beyond consciousness. The person in a state of samādhi is fully conscious and alert.

All creation is Brahman. The sādhaka is tranquil and worships it as that from which he came forth, as that in which he breathes, as that into which he will be dissolved. The soul within the heart is smaller than the smallest seed, yet greater than the sky, containing all works, all desires. Into this the sādhaka enters. Then there remains no sense of 'I' or 'mine' as the working of the body, the mind and the intellect have stopped as if one is in deep sleep. The sādhaka has attained true Yoga; there is only the experience of consciousness, truth and unutterable joy. There is a peace that passeth all understanding. The mind cannot find words to describe the state and the tongue fails to utter them. Comparing the experience of samādhi with other experiences, the sages say: 'Neti! Neti!' – 'It is not this! It is not this!' The state can only be expressed by profound silence. The yogi has departed from the material world and is merged in the Eternal. There is then no duality between the knower and the known for they are merged like camphor and the flame.

There wells up from within the heart of the yogi the Song of the Soul, sung by Śankarāchārya in his *Ātma Ṣaṭkam*.

Song of the Soul

I am neither ego nor reason, I am neither mind nor thought,
I cannot be heard nor cast into words, nor by smell nor sight ever caught:
In light and wind I am not found, nor yet in earth and sky –
Consciousness and joy incarnate, Bliss of the Blissful am I.

I have no name, I have no life, I breathe no vital air,
No elements have moulded me, no bodily sheath is my lair:
I have no speech, no hands and feet, nor means of evolution –
Consciousness and joy am I, and Bliss in dissolution.

I cast aside hatred and passion, I conquered delusion and greed;
No touch of pride caressed me, so envy never did breed:
Beyond all faiths, past reach of wealth, past freedom, past desire,
Consciousness and joy am I, and Bliss is my attire.

Virtue and vice, or pleasure and pain are not my heritage,
Nor sacred texts, nor offerings, nor prayer, nor pilgrimage:
I am neither food, nor eating, nor yet the eater am I –
Consciousness and joy incarnate, Bliss of the Blissful am I.

I have no misgiving of death, no chasms of race divide me,
No parent ever called me child, no bond of birth ever tied me:
I am neither disciple nor master, I have no kin, no friend –
Consciousness and joy am I, and merging in Bliss is my end.

Neither knowable, knowledge, nor knower am I, formless is my form,
I dwell within the senses but they are not my home:
Ever serenely balanced, I am neither free nor bound –
Consciousness and joy am I, and Bliss is where I am found.

Part II
Yogāsanas

Hints, Cautions, Technique and Effects

(After the name of each āsana, there is a number with an asterisk. These numbers before an asterisk indicate the intensity of the āsana; the lower the number, the easier the āsana, the higher the number, the more difficult the āsana.)

Yogāsanas

Hints and Cautions for the Practice of Āsanas

The requisites

1 Without firm foundations a house cannot stand. Without the practice of the principles of yama and niyama, which lay down firm foundations for building character, there cannot be an integrated personality. Practice of āsanas without the backing of yama and niyama is mere acrobatics.

2 The qualities demanded from an aspirant are discipline, faith, tenacity and perseverance to practice regularly without interruptions.

Cleanliness and food

3. Before starting to practise āsanas, the bladder should be emptied and the bowels evacuated. Topsy-turvy poses help bowel movements. If the student is constipated or it is not possible to evacuate the bowels before the practice of āsanas, start with Śīrṣāsana and Sarvāngāsana and their variations. Attempt other āsanas only after evacuation. Never practice advanced āsanas without having first evacuated the bowels.

Bath

4. Āsanas come easier after taking a bath. After doing them, the body feels sticky due to perspiration and it is desirable to bathe some fifteen minutes later. Taking a bath or a shower both before and after practising āsanas refreshes the body and mind.

Food

5. Āsanas should preferably be done on an empty stomach. If this is difficult, a cup of tea or coffee, cocoa or milk may be taken before doing them. They may be practised without

discomfort one hour after a very light meal. Allow at least four hours to elapse after a heavy meal before starting the practice. Food may be taken half an hour after completing the āsanas.

Time

6. The best time to practise is either early in the morning or late in the evening. In the morning āsanas do not come easily as the body is stiff. The mind, however, is still fresh but its alertness and determination diminish as time goes by. The stiffness of the body is conquered by regular practice and one is able to do the āsanas well. In the evening, the body moves more freely than in the mornings, and the āsanas come better and with greater ease. Practice in the morning makes one work better in one's vocation. In the evening it removes the fatigue of the day's strain and makes one fresh and calm. Do all the āsanas in the morning and stimulative āsanas (like Śīrṣāsana, Sarvāṅgāsana and their variations and Paśchimottānāsana) should be practised in the evening.

Sun

7. Do not practise āsanas after being out in the hot sun for several hours.

Place

8. They should be done in a clean airy place, free from insects and noise.

9. Do not do them on the bare floor or on an uneven place, but on a folded blanket laid on a level floor.

Caution

10. No undue strain should be felt in the facial muscles, ears and eyes or in breathing during the practice.

Closing of the eyes

11. In the beginning, keep the eyes open. Then you will know what you are doing and where you go wrong. If you shut your eyes you will not be able to watch the requisite

movements of the body or even the direction in which you are doing the pose. You can keep your eyes closed only when you are perfect in a particular āsana for only then will you be able to adjust the bodily movements and feel the correct stretches.

Mirror

12. If you are doing the āsanas in front of a mirror, keep it perpendicular to the floor and let it come down to ground level, for otherwise the poses will look slanting due to the angle of the mirror. You will not be able to observe the movements of placing the head and shoulders in the topsy-turvy poses unless the mirror reaches down to the floor. Use a mirror without a frame.

The Brain

13. During the practice of āsanas, it is the body alone which should be active while the brain should remain passive, watchful and alert. If they are done with the brain, then you will not be able to see your own mistakes.

Breathing

14. In all the āsanas, breathing should be done through the nostrils only and not through the mouth.

15. Do not restrain the breath while in the process of the āsana or while staying in it. Follow the instructions regarding breathing given in the technique sections of the various āsanas as described hereafter.

Śavāsana

16. After completing the practice of āsanas always lie down in Śavāsana for at least 10 to 15 minutes, as this will remove fatigue.

Āsanas and Prāṇāyāma

17. Read carefully the hints and cautions for the practice of prāṇāyāma before attempting it (see Part III). Prāṇāyāma may be done either very early in the morning before the āsanas or in the evening after completing them. If early in the

morning, prāṇāyāma may be done first for 15 to 30 minutes: then a few minutes of Śavāsana, and after allowing some time to elapse, during which one may be engaged in normal activities, practise āsanas. If, however, these are done in the evening, allow at least half an hour to elapse before sitting for prāṇāyāma.

Special provisions for persons suffering from dizziness or blood· pressure

18. Do not start with Śīrṣāsana and Sarvāngāsana if you suffer from dizziness or high blood pressure. First practise Paśchimottānāsana Uttānāsana, and Adho Mukha Śvānāsana before attempting topsy-turvy poses like Śīrṣāsana and Sarvāngāsana and after doing these poses repeat Paśchimottānāsana, Adho Mukha Śvānāsana and Uttānāsana in that order

19. All forward bending poses are beneficial for persons suffering from either high or low blood pressure.

Special warning for persons affected from pus in the ears or displaced retina

20. Those suffering from pus in the ears or displacement of the retina should not attempt topsy-turvy poses.

Special provisions for women

21. *Menstruation:* Avoid āsanas during the menstrual period. But if the flow is in excess of normal, Upaviṣṭha Koṇāsana, Baddha Koṇāsana, Vīrāsana, Jānu Śīrṣāsana, Paśchimottānāsana and Uttānāsana will be beneficial. On no account stand on your head nor perform sarvāngāsana, during the menstrual period.

Pregnancy

22. All the āsanas can be practised during the first three months of pregnancy. All the standing poses and the forward bending āsanas may be done with mild movements, for at this time the spine should be made strong and elastic and no pressure be felt on the abdomen. Baddha Koṇāsana and

Upaviṣṭha Koṇāsana may be practised throughout pregnancy at any time of the day (even after meals, but not forward bending immediately after meals) as these two āsanas will strengthen the pelvic muscles and the small of the back and also reduce labour pains considerably. Prāṇāyāma without retention (kumbhaka) may be practised throughout pregnancy, as regular deep breathing will help considerably during labour.

After delivery

23. No āsanas should be done during the first month after delivery. Thereafter they may be practised mildly. Gradually increase the course as mentioned in the Appendix. Three months after delivery all āsanas may be practised with comfort.

Effects of āsanas

24. Faulty practice causes discomfort and uneasiness within a few days. This is sufficient to show that one is going wrong. If you cannot find the fault yourself, it is better to approach a person who has practised well and get his guidance.

25. The right method of doing āsanas brings lightness and an exhilarating feeling in the body as well as in the mind and a feeling of oneness of body, mind and soul.

26. Continuous practice will change the outlook of the practiser. He will discipline himself in food, sex, cleanliness and character and will become a new man.

27. When one has mastered an āsana, it comes with effortless ease and causes no discomfort. The bodily movements become graceful. While performing āsanas, the student's body assumes numerous forms of life found in creation – from the lowliest insect to the most perfect sage – and he learns that in all these there breathes the same Universal Spirit – the Spirit of God. He looks within himself while practising and feels the presence of God in different āsanas which he does with a sense of surrender unto the feet of the LORD.

ĀSANAS

1. *Tāḍāsana* (also called Samasthiti) One* (Plate 1)

Tāḍa means a mountain. Sama means upright, straight, unmoved. Sthiti is standing still, steadiness. Tāḍāsana therefore implies a pose where one stands firm and erect as a mountain. This is the basic standing pose.

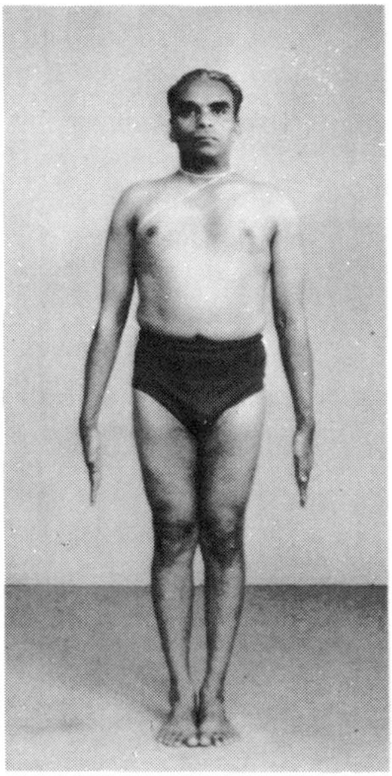

1

Technique

1. Stand erect with the feet together, the heels and big toes touching each other. Rest the heads of metatarsals on the floor and stretch all the toes flat on the floor.

2. Tighten the knees and pull the knee-caps up, contract the hips and pull up the muscles at the back of the thighs.

3. Keep the stomach in, chest forward, spine stretched up and the neck straight.

4. Do not bear the weight of the body either on the heels or the toes, but distribute it evenly on them both.

5. Ideally in Tāḍāsana the arms are stretched out over the head, but for the sake of convenience, one can place them by the side of the thighs. In this case, keep the arms parallel with the body. The fingers together and pointings downwards. Each of the standing poses described below can then be followed easily, starting with the pupil standing in Tāḍāsana with palms by the side of the thighs.

Effects

People do not pay attention to the correct method of standing. Some stand with the body weight thrown only on one leg, or with one leg turned completely sideways. Others bear all the weight on the heels, or on the inner or outer edges of the feet. This can be noticed by watching where the soles and heels of the shoes wear out. Owing to our faulty method of standing and not distributing the body weight evenly on the feet, we acquire specific deformities which hamper spinal elasticity. Even if the feet are kept apart, it is better to keep the heel and toe in a line parallel to the median plane and not at an angle. By this method, the hips are contracted, the abdomen is pulled in and the chest is brought forward. One feels light in body and the mind acquires agility. If we stand with the body weight thrown only on the heels, we feel the centre of gravity changing; the hips become loose, the abdomen protrudes, the body hangs back and the spine feels the strain and consequently we soon feel fatigued and the mind becomes dull. It is therefore essential to master the art of standing correctly.

2. *Utthita Trikoṇāsana* Three* (Plates 3 and 4)

Utthita means extended, stretched. Trikoṇa (tri=three; koṇa=angle) is a triangle. This standing āsana is the extended triangle pose.

Technique

1. Stand in Tāḍāsana. (Plate 1)

2. Inhale deeply and with a jump spread apart the legs sideways 3 to $3\frac{1}{2}$ feet. Raise the arms sideways, in line with the shoulders, palms facing down. Keep the arms parallel to the floor. (Plate 2)

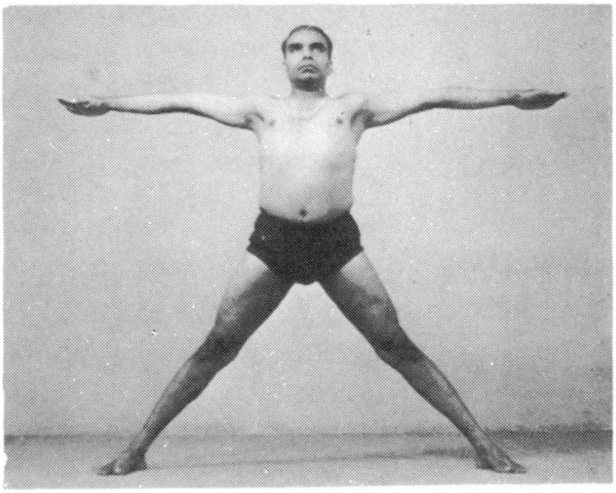

2

3. Turn the right foot sideways 90 degrees to the right. Turn the left foot slightly to the right, keeping the left leg stretched from the inside and tightened at the knee.

4. Exhale, bend the trunk sideways to the right, bringing the right palm near the right angle. If possible, the right palm should rest completely on the floor. (Plates 3 and 4)

5. Stretch the left arm up (as in the illustration), bringing it in line with the right shoulder and extend the trunk. The back of the legs, the back of the chest and the hips should be in line. Gaze at the thumb of the outstretched left hand. Keep the right knee locked tight by pulling up the knee-cap and keep the right knee facing the toes.

6. Remain in this position from half a minute to a minute, breathing deeply and evenly. Then lift the right palm from the floor. Inhale and return to position 2 above.

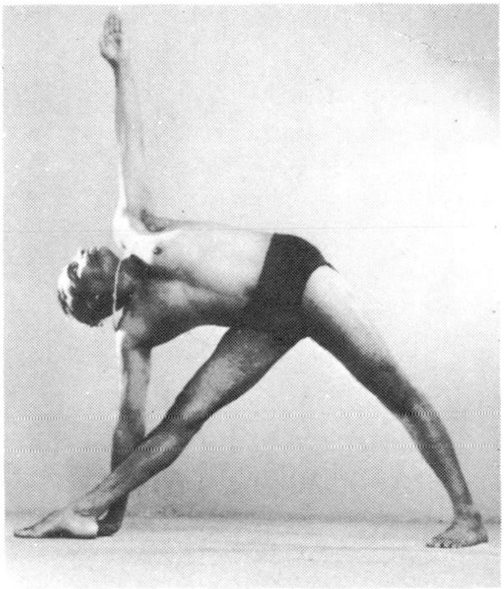

3

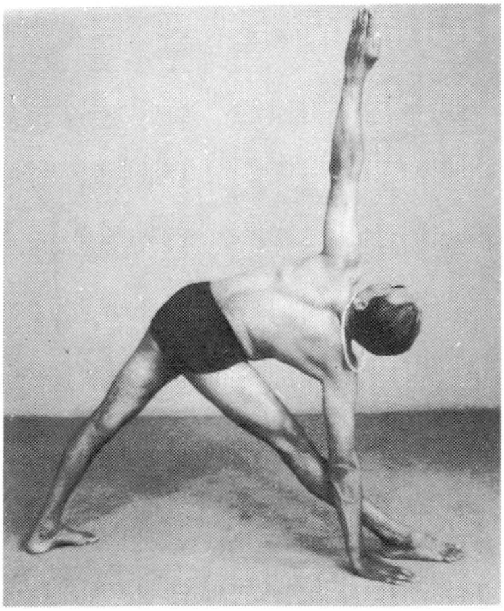

4

7. Now, turn the left foot sideways 90 degrees to the left, turn the right foot slightly to the left, keep both knees tight and continue from position 2 to 6, reversing all processes. Inhale and come to position 2. Hold the posture for the same length of time on the left side.

8. Exhale, and jump, coming back to Tāḍāsana. (Plate 1)

Effects

This āsana tones up the leg muscles, removes stiffness in the legs and hips, corrects any minor deformity in the legs and allows them to develop evenly. It relieves backaches and neck sprains, strengthens the ankles and develops the chest.

3. *Utthita Pārśvakoṇāsana* Four* (Plates 5 and 6)

Pārśva means side or flank. Koṇa is an angle. This is the extended lateral angle pose.

Technique

1. Stand in Tāḍāsana. (Plate 1.) Take a deep inhalation and with a jump spread the legs apart sideways 4 to 4½ feet. Raise the arms sideways, in line with the shoulders, palms facing down. (Plate 2)

2. While exhaling slowly, turn the right foot sideways 90 degrees to the right, and the left foot slightly to the right, keeping the left leg stretched out and tightened at the knee. Bend the right leg at the knee until the thigh and the calf form a right angle and the right thigh is parallel to the floor.

3. Place the right palm on the floor by the side of the right foot, the right armpit covering and touching the outer side of the right knee. Stretch the left arm out over the left ear. Keep the head up. (Plates 5 and 6)

4. Tighten the loins and stretch the hamstrings. The chest, the hips and the legs should be in a line and in order to achieve this, move the chest up and back. Stretch every part of the body, concentrating on the back portion of the whole

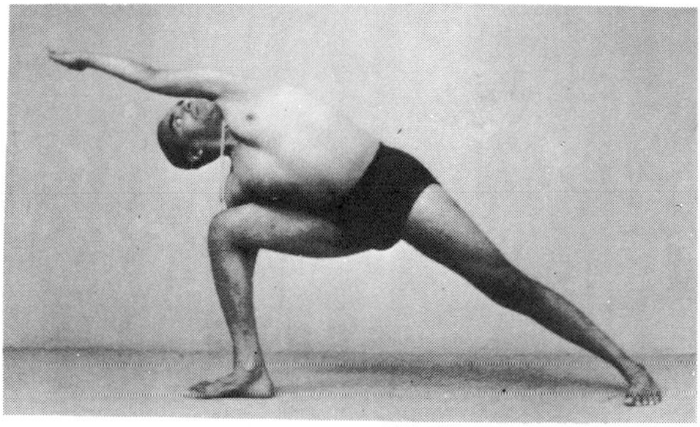

5

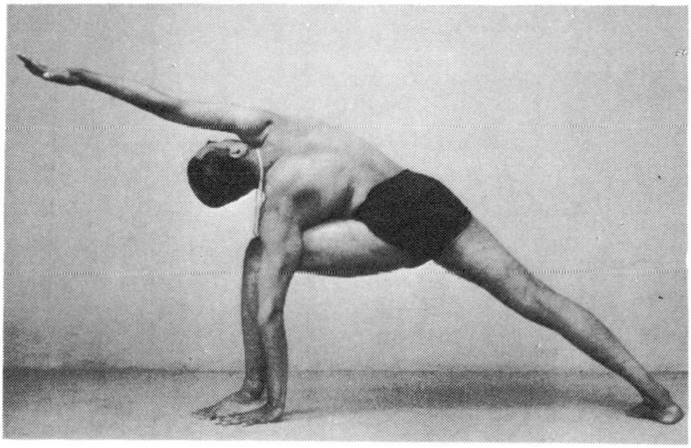

6

body, specially the spine. Stretch the spine until all the vertebrae and ribs move and there is a feeling that even the skin is being stretched and pulled.

5. Remain in this pose from half a minute to a minute, breathing deeply and evenly. Inhale and lift the right palm from the floor.

6. Inhale, straighten the right leg and raise the arms as in position 1.

7. Continue with exhalation as in positions 2 to 5, reversing all processes, on the left side.

8. Exhale and jump back to Tāḍāsana. (Plate 1)

Effects

This āsana tones up the ankles, knees and thighs. It corrects defects in the calves and thighs, develops the chest and reduces fat round the waist and hips and relieves sciatic and arthritic pains. It also increases peristaltic activity and aids elimination.

4. *Vīrabhadrāsana I* Three* (Plate 9)

Dakṣa once celebrated a great sacrifice, but he did not invite his daughter Satī nor her husband Śiva, the chief of the gods. Satī, however, went to the sacrifice, but being greatly humiliated and insulted threw herself into the fire and perished. When Śiva heard this he was gravely provoked, tore a hair from his matted locks and threw it to the ground. A powerful hero named Vīrabhadra rose up and awaited his orders. He was told to lead Śiva's army against Dakṣa and destroy his sacrifice. Vīrabhadra and his army appeared in the midst of Dakṣa's assembly like a hurricane and destroyed the sacrifice, routed the other gods and priests and beheaded Dakṣa. Śiva in grief for Satī withdrew to Kailās and plunged into meditation. Satī was born again as Umā in the house of Himālaya. She strove once more for the love of Śiva and ultimately won his heart. The story is told by Kālidāsa in his great poem *Kumāra saṁbhava* (The Birth of the War-Lord). This āsana is dedicated to the powerful hero created by Śiva from his matted hair.

Technique

1. Stand in Tāḍāsana. (Plate 1)

2. Raise both arms above the head; stretch up and join the palms. (Plate 7)

3. Take a deep inhalation and with a jump spread the legs apart sideways 4 to $4\frac{1}{2}$ feet.

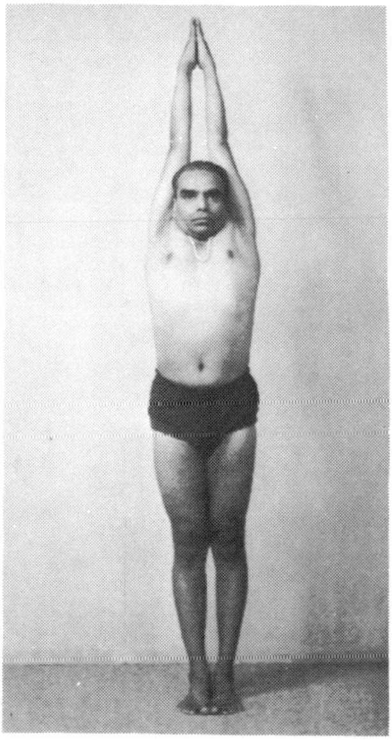

7

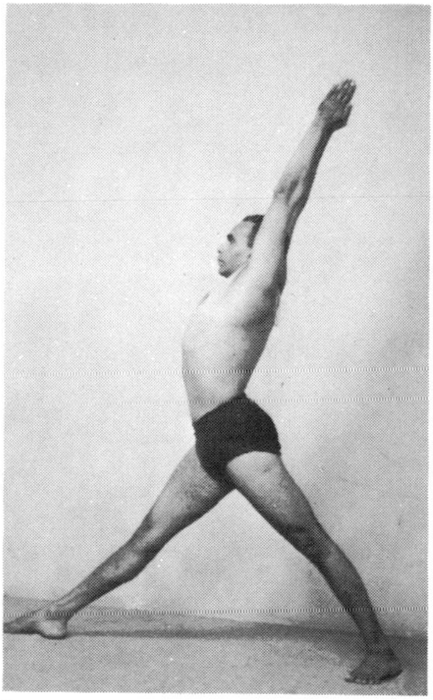

8

4. Exhale, turn to the right. Simultaneously turn the right foot 90 degrees to the right and the left foot slightly to the right. (Plate 8.) Flex the right knee till the right thigh is parallel to the floor and the right shin perpendicular to the floor, forming a right angle between the right thigh and the right calf. The bent knee should not extend beyond the ankle, but should be in line with the heel.

5. Stretch out the left leg and tighten at the knee.

6. The face, chest and right knee should face the same way as the right foot, as illustrated. Throw the head up, stretch the spine from the coccyx and gaze at the joined palms. (Plate 9)

7. Hold the pose from 20 seconds to half a minute with normal breathing.

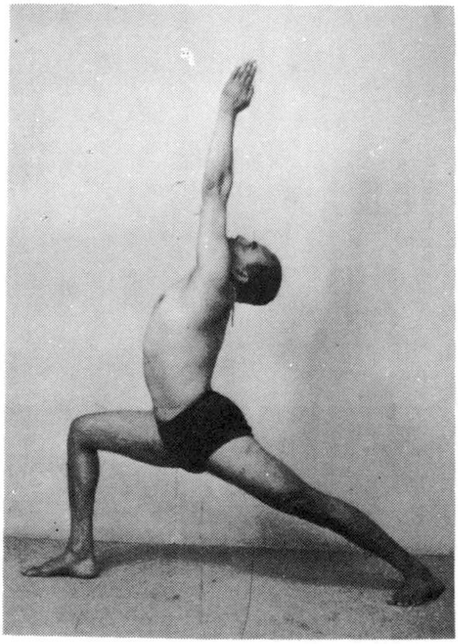

9

8. Repeat on the left side as in positions 4 to 6, reversing all processes.

9. Exhale and jump back to Tāḍāsana. (Plate 1)

***All standing poses are strenuous, this pose in particular. It should not be tried by persons with a weak heart. Even people who are fairly strong should not stay long in this āsana.

Effects
In this pose the chest is fully expanded and this helps deep breathing. It relieves stiffness in shoulders and back, tones up the ankles and knees and cures stiffness of the neck. It also reduces fat round the hips.

5. *Vīrabhadrāsana II* One* (Plate 10)

Technique

1. Stand in Tāḍāsana. (Plate 1)

2. Take a deep inhalation, and with a jump spread the legs apart sideways 4 to 4½ feet. Raise the arms sideways in line with the shoulders, palms facing down. (Plate 2)

3. Turn the right foot sideways 90 degrees to the right and the left foot slightly to the right, keeping the left leg stretched out and tightened at the knee. Stretch the hamstring muscles of the left leg.

4. Exhale and bend the right knee till the right thigh is parallel to the floor, keeping the right shin perpendicular to the floor, thus forming a right angle between the right thigh and the right calf. The bent knee should not extend beyond the ankle, but should be in line with the heel. (Plate 10)

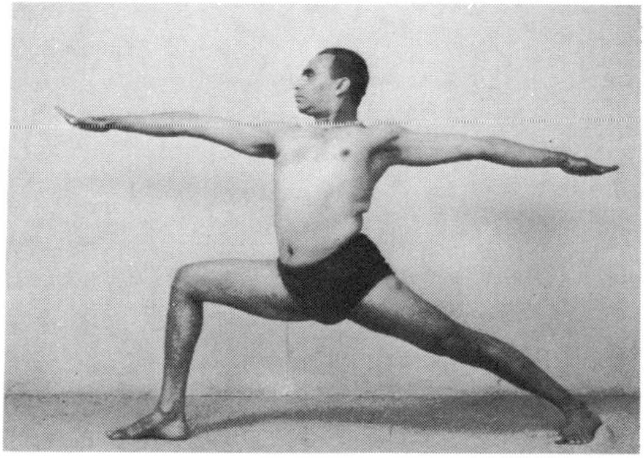

10

5. Stretch out the hands sideways, as though two persons are pulling you from opposite ends.

6. Turn the face to the right and gaze at the right palm. Stretch the back muscles of the left leg fully. The back of the legs, the dorsal region and the hips should be in one line.

7. Stay in the pose from 20 seconds to half a minute with deep breathing. Inhale and return to position 2.

8. Turn the left foot sideways 90 degrees to the left and the right foot slightly to the left, flex the left knee and continue from positions 3 to 6 on the left side, reversing all processes.

9. Inhale, again come back to position 2. Exhale and jump back to Tāḍāsana. (Plate 1)

Effects

Through this pose the leg muscles become shapely and stronger. It relieves cramp in the calf and thigh muscles, brings elasticity to the leg and back muscles and also tones the abdominal organs.

Mastery of the standing poses prepares the pupil for the advanced poses in forward bending, which can then be acquired with ease.

6. *Pārśvōttānāsana* Six* (Plate 13)

Pārśva means side or flank. Uttāna (ut=intense, and tān=to extend, stretch, lengthen) means an intense stretch. The name implies a pose in which the side of the chest is stretched intensely.

Technique

1. Stand in Tāḍāsana. (Plate 1.) Inhale deeply and stretch the body forward.

2. Join the palms behind the back and draw the shoulders and elbows back.

3. Exhale, turn the wrists and bring both palms up above the middle of the back of the chest, the fingers at the level of the shoulderblades. You are doing 'namaste' (the Indian gesture of respect by folding the hands) with your hands behind your back. (Plate 11)

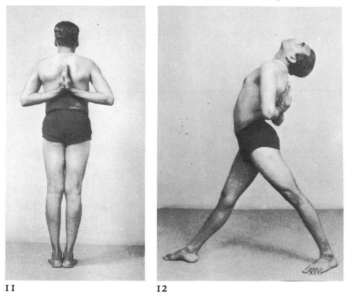

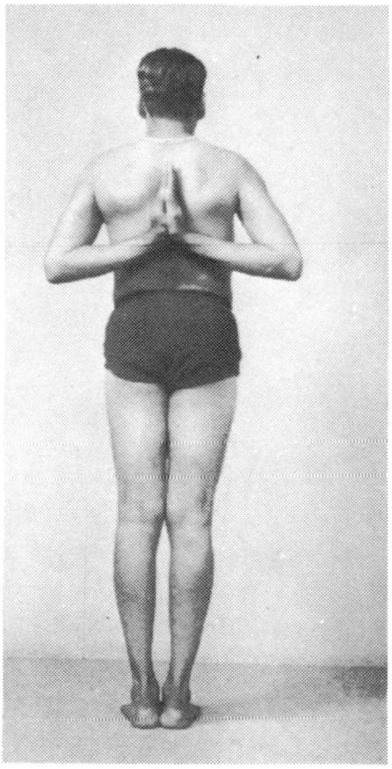

11

12

4. Inhale and with a jump spread the legs apart sideways 3 to $3\frac{1}{2}$ feet. Stay in this position and exhale.

5. Inhale and turn the trunk to the right. Turn the right foot 90 degrees sideways to the right keeping the toes and heel in a line with the trunk; turn the left foot with the leg 75 to 80 degrees to the right and keep the left foot stretched out and the leg tightened at the knee. Throw the head back. (Plate 12)

6. Exhale, bend the trunk forward and rest the head on the right knee. Stretch the back and gradually extend the neck until the nose, then the lips and lastly the chin touch and then rest beyond the right knee. (Plate 13.) Tighten both the legs by pulling the knee-caps up.

7. Stay in the pose from 20 seconds to half a minute with normal breathing. Then slowly move the head and trunk

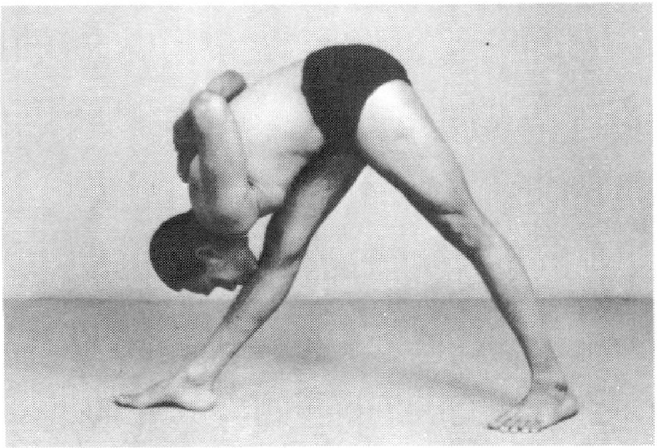

13

towards the left knee by swinging the trunk round the hips. At the same time turn the left foot 90 degrees towards the left and the right foot 75 to 80 degrees to the left. Now raise the trunk and head as far back as you can, without bending the right leg. This movement should be done with one inhalation.

8. Exhale, bend the trunk forward, rest the head on the left knee and gradually extend the chin beyond the left knee by stretching the neck as in position 6.

9. After holding the pose from 20 seconds to half a minute with normal breathing, inhale, move the head to the centre and the feet to their original position so that the toes point forward. Then raise the trunk up.

10. Exhale and jump back to Tāḍāsana (Plate 1), releasing the hands from the back.

11. If you cannot fold the hands together behind the back, just grip the right wrist and follow the above technique. (Plate 14)

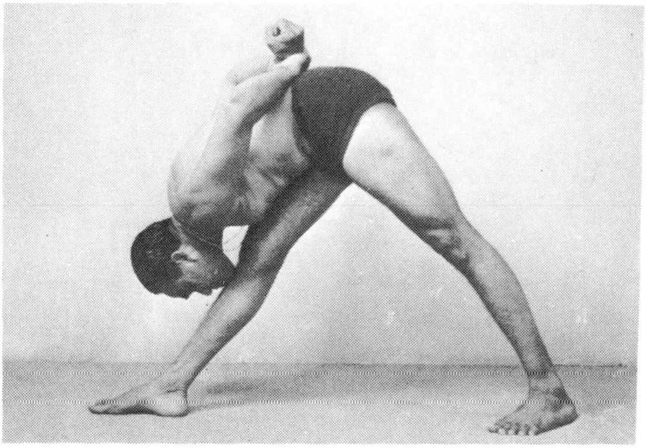

14

Effects
This āsana relieves stiffness in the legs and hip muscles and makes the hip joints and spine elastic. While the head is resting on the knees, the abdominal organs are contracted and toned. The wrists move freely and any stiffness there disappears. The posture also corrects round and drooping shoulders. In the correct pose, the shoulders are drawn well back and this makes deep breathing easier.

7. *Prasārita Pādōttānāsana I* Four* (Plates 17 and 18)
Prasārita means expanded, spread, extended. Pāda means a foot. The pose is one where the expanded legs are stretched intensely.

Technique
1. Stand in Tāḍāsana. (Plate 1)

2. Inhale, place the hands on the waist and spread the legs apart 4½ to 5 feet. (Plate 15)

3. Tighten the legs by drawing up the knee-caps. Exhale, and place the palms on the floor in line with the shoulders between the feet. (Plate 16)

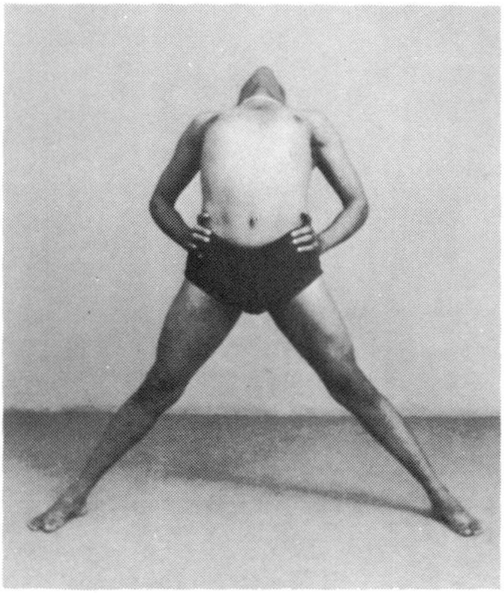

15

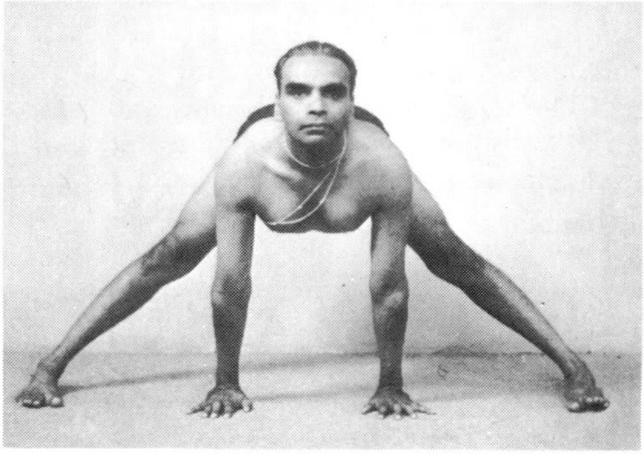

16

4. Inhale and raise the head up, keeping the back concave.

5. Exhale, bend the elbows and rest the crown of the head on the floor, keeping the weight of the body on the legs. (Plates 17 and 18.) Do not throw the body weight on the head. Both feet, both palms and the head should be in a straight line.

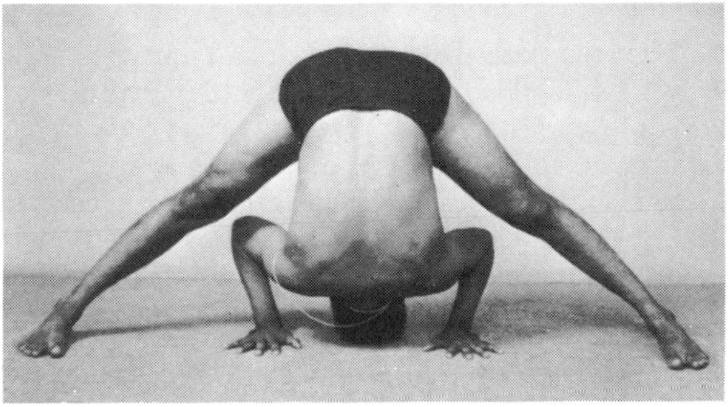

17

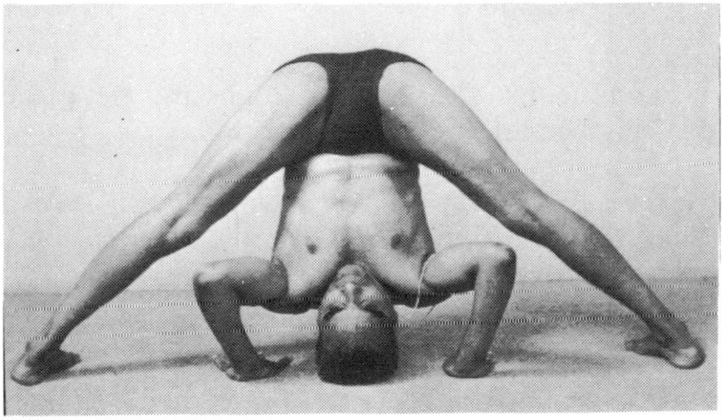

18

6. Stay in the pose for half a minute, breathing deeply and evenly.

7. Inhale, raise the head from the floor and straighten the arms at the elbows. Keep the head well up by making the back concave as in position 4. (Plate 16)

8. Exhale and stand as in position 2. (Plate 15)

9. Jump back to Tāḍāsana. (Plate 1)

Effects

In this pose the hamstring and abductor muscles are fully developed, while blood is made to flow to the trunk and the head. People who cannot do Śīrṣāsana (Plate 90) can benefit from this pose, which increases digestive powers.

All the standing poses described above are necessary for beginners. As the pupil advances he attains better flexibility and then the standing poses can be dispensed with, though it is advisable to do them once a week. All these standing poses help to reduce the body weight.

8. *Uṣṭrāsana* Three* (Plate 20)
Uṣṭra means a camel.

Technique

1. Kneel on the floor, keeping the thighs and feet together, toes pointing back and resting on the floor.

2. Rest the palms on the hips. Stretch the thighs, curve the spine back and extend the ribs. (Plate 19)

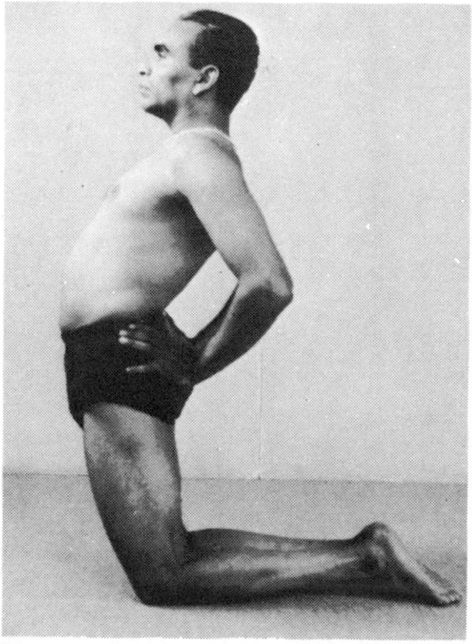

19

3. Exhale, place the right palm over the right heel and the left palm over the left heel. If possible, place the palms on the soles of the feet.

4. Press the feet with the palms, throw the head back and push the spine towards the thighs, which should be kept perpendicular to the floor.

5. Contract the buttocks and stretch the dorsal and the coccyx regions of the spine still further, keeping the neck stretched back. (Plate 20)

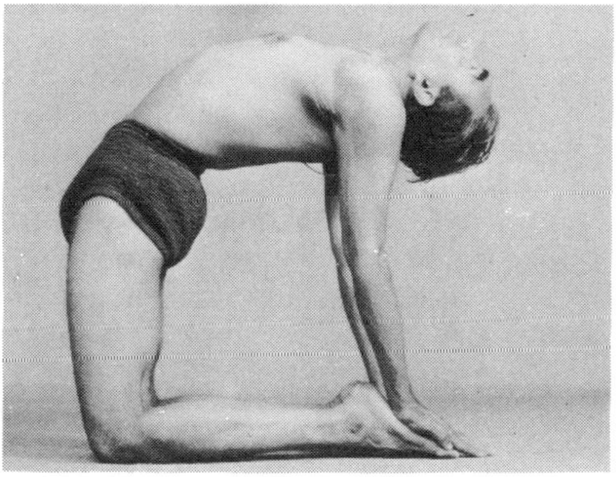

20

6. Remains in this position for about half a minute with normal breathing.

7. Release the hands one by one and rest them on the hips. (Plate 19) Then sit on the floor and relax.

Effects

People with drooping shoulders and hunched backs will benefit by this āsana

The whole spine is stretched back and is toned. This pose can be tried conveniently by the elderly and even by persons with spinal injury.

9. *Pādānguṣṭhāsana* Three* (Plate 22)

Pāda means the foot. Anguṣṭha is the big toe. This posture is done by standing and catching the big toes.

Technique

1. Stand in Tāḍāsana. (Plate 1) Spread the legs a foot apart.

2. Exhale, bend forward and hold the big toes between the thumbs and the first two fingers, so that the palms face each other. Hold them tight. (Plate 21)

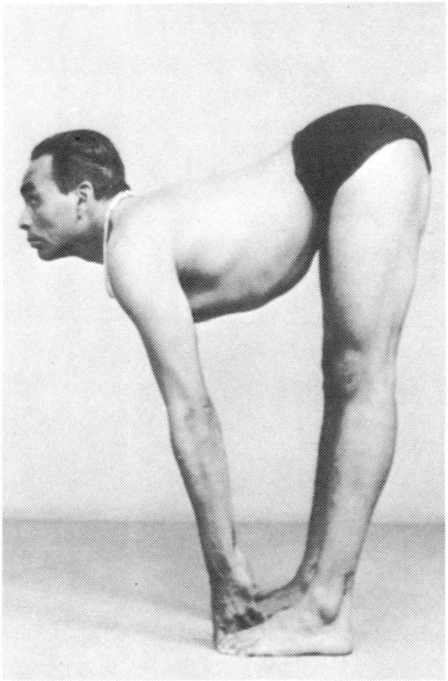

21

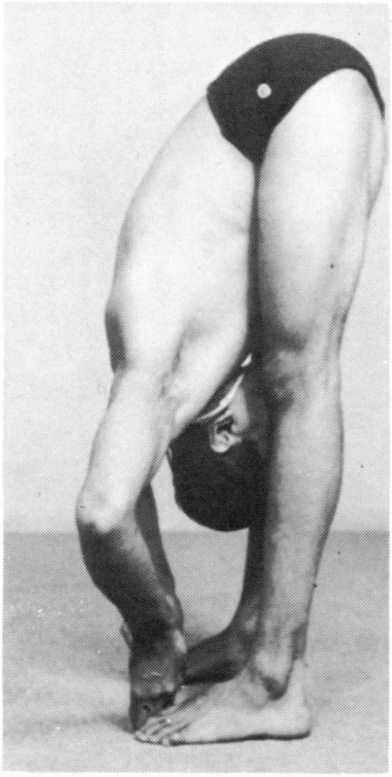

22

3. Keep the head up, stretch the diaphragm towards the chest and make the back as concave as possible. Instead of stretching down from the shoulders, bend forward from the pelvic region to get the concave shape of the back from the coccyx.

4. Keep the legs stiff and do not slacken the grip at the knees and toes. Stretch the shoulder-blades also. Take one or two breaths in this position.

5. Now exhale, and bring the head in between the knees by tightening and pulling the toes without lifting them off the floor. (Plate 22) Remain in this pose for about 20 seconds, maintaining normal breathing.

6. Inhale, come to position 2 (Plate 21), release the toes and stand up. Return to Tāḍāsana. (Plate 1)

10. *Pādahastāsana* Six* (Plate 24)
Pāda means the foot. Hasta means the hand. This posture is done by bending forward and standing on one's hands.

Technique
1. Stand in Tāḍāsana. (Plate 1) Spread the legs a foot apart.

2. Exhale, bend forward and without bending the legs at the knees insert the hands under the feet so that the palms touch the soles. (Plate 23)

3. Keep the head up and make the back as concave as possible. Do not slacken the grip at the knees and take a few breaths in this position.

4. Now exhale, and move the head in between the knees by bending the elbows and pulling the feet up from the palms. (Plate 24) Stay in the pose for about 20 seconds with normal breathing.

5. Inhale, raise the head and come back to position 2 (Plate 23), with the head well up. Take two breaths.

6. Inhale, stand up and return to Tāḍāsana. (Plate 1)

Effects of Pādānguṣṭhāsana and Pādahastāsana
The second āsana is more strenuous than the first, but the

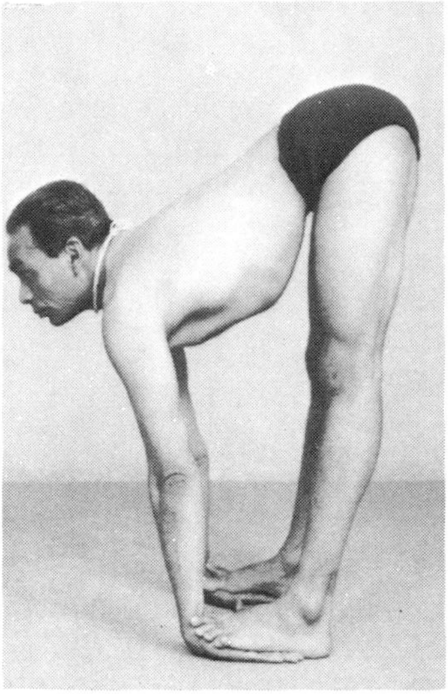

23

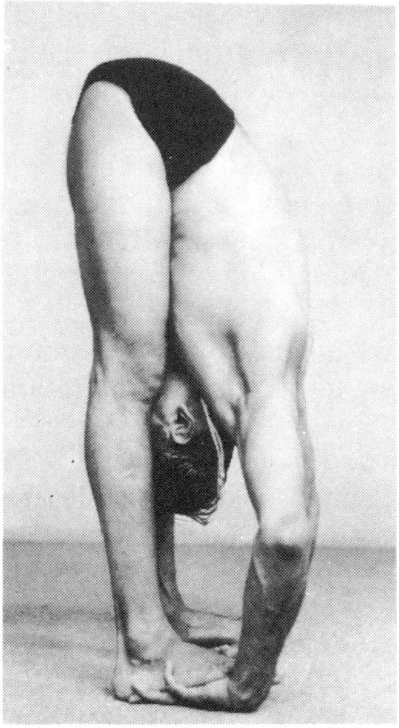

24

effects of both are the same. The abdominal organs are toned and digestive juices increase, while the liver and spleen are activated. Persons suffering from a bloating sensation in the abdomen or from gastric troubles will benefit by practising these two āsanas.

Slipped spinal discs can only be adjusted in the concave back position as in Plates 21 and 23. Do not bring the head in between the knees if you have a displaced disc. I have experimented with persons suffering from slipped discs and the concave back position proved a boon to them. It is imperative to get guidance from a guru (master) before trying this pose, because it may not be possible to achieve the concave back position immediately. One has to master other minor poses before attempting this one.

11. *Uttānāsana* Eight* (Plate 25)

Ut is a particle indicating deliberation. intensity. The verb tān means to stretch, extend, lengthen out. In this āsana, the spine is given a deliberate and an intense stretch.

Technique

1. Stand in Tāḍāsana (Plate 1), keeping the knees tight.

2. Exhale, bend forward and place the fingers on the floor. Then place the palms on the floor by the side of the feet, behind the heels. Do not bend the legs at the knees.

3. Try to hold the head up and stretch the spine. Move the hips a little forward towards the head so as to bring the legs perpendicular to the floor.

4. Remain in this position and take two deep breaths.

5. Exhale, move the trunk closer to the legs and rest the head on the knees. (Plate 25)

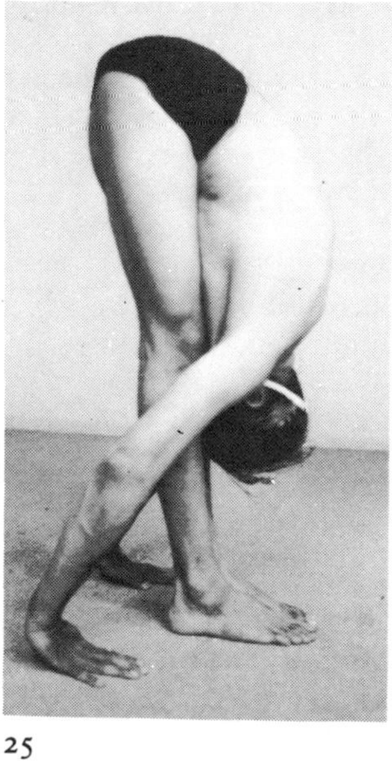

25

6. Do not slacken the grip at the knees, but pull the kneecaps well up. Hold this position for a minute with deep and even breathing.

7. Inhale and raise the head from the knees, but without lifting the palms from the floor as in position 3.

8. After two breaths, take a deep inhalation, lift the hands from the floor and come back to Tāḍāsana. (Plate 1)

Effects

This āsana cures stomach pains and tones the liver, the spleen and the kidneys. It also relieves stomach pain during menstrual periods. The heart beats are slowed down and the spinal nerves rejuvenated. Any depression felt in the mind is removed if one holds the pose for two minutes or more. The posture is a boon to people who get excited quickly, as it soothes the brain cells. After finishing the āsana, one feels calm and cool, the eyes start to glow and the mind feels at peace.

Persons who feel heaviness in the head, flushing or any discomfort while attempting Śīrṣāsana (Plate 90), should do Uttānāsana first; then they will be able to do Śīrsāsana (the head stand) with comfort and ease.

12. *Śalabhāsana* One* (Plate 26)

Śalabhā means a locust. The pose resembles that of a locust resting on the ground, hence the name.

Technique

1. Lie full length on the floor on the stomach, face downwards. Stretch the arms back.

2. Exhale, lift the head, chest and legs off the floor simultaneously as high as possible. The hands should not be placed and the ribs should not rest on the floor. Only the abdominal front portion of the body rests on the floor and bears the weight of the body. (Plate 26)

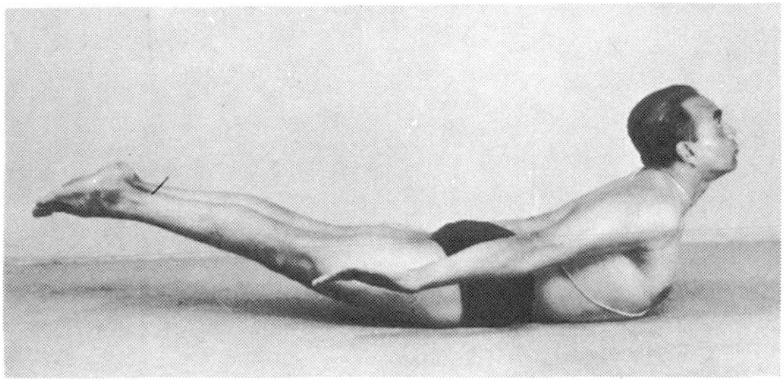

26

3. Contract the buttocks and stretch the thigh muscles. Keep both legs fully extended and straight, touching at the thighs, knees and ankles.

4. Do not bear the weight of the body on the hands but stretch them back to exercise the upper portion of the back muscles.

5. Stay in the position as long as you can with normal breathing.

6. In the beginning it is difficult to lift the chest and the legs off the floor, but this becomes easier as the abdominal muscles grow stronger.

Effects
The pose aids digestion and relieves gastric troubles and flatulence. Since the spine is stretched back it becomes elastic and the pose relieves pain in the sacral and lumbar regions. In my experience, persons suffering from slipped discs have benefited by regular practice of this āsana without recourse to enforced rest or surgical treatment. The bladder and the prostate gland also benefit from the exercise and remain healthy.

A variation of the pose may also be tried to relieve aches in the lower part of the back. Here, the legs are bent at the knees and the thighs are kept apart while the shins are kept

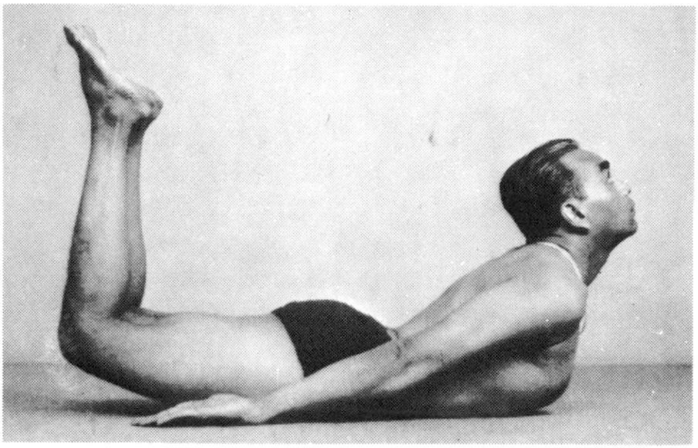

27

perpendicular to the floor. Then with an exhalation, the thighs are lifted off the floor and brought closer together until the knees touch, the shins still being kept perpendicular. (Plate 27)

13. *Dhanurāsana* Four* (Plate 28)
Dhanu means a bow. The hands here are used like a bow-string to pull the head, trunk and legs up and the posture resembles a bent bow.

Technique

1. Lie full length on the floor on the stomach, face downwards.

2. Exhale and bend the knees. Stretch the arms back and hold the left ankle with the left hand and the right ankle with the right hand. Take two breaths.

3. Now exhale completely and pull the legs up by raising the knees above the floor, and simultaneously lift the chest off the floor. The arms and hands act like a bow-string to tauten the body like a bent bow. (Plate 28)

4. Lift up the head and pull it as far back as possible. Do not

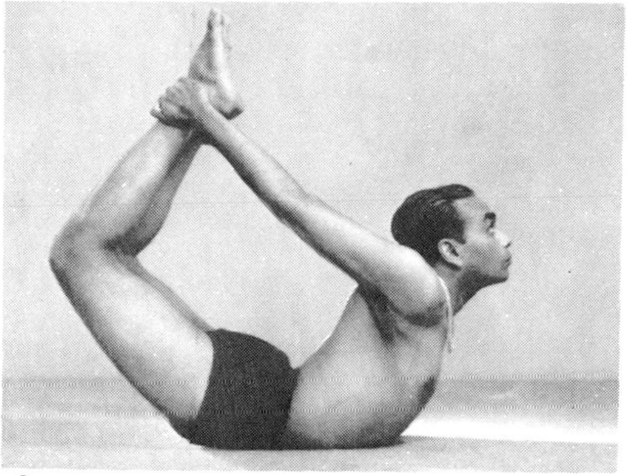

28

rest either the ribs or the pelvic bones on the floor. Only the abdomen bears the weight of the body on the floor.

5. While raising the legs do not join them at the knees, for then the legs will not be lifted high enough. After the full stretch upwards has been achieved, join together the thighs, the knees and the ankles.

6. Since the abdomen is extended, the breathing will be fast, but do not worry about it. Stay in the pose to your capacity from 20 seconds to one minute.

7. Then, with an exhalation, release the ankles, stretch the legs straight, bring the head and the legs back to the floor and relax.

Effects
In this posture the spine is stretched back. Elderly people do not normally do this, so their spines get rigid. This āsana brings back elasticity to the spine and tones the abdominal organs. In my experience, persons suffering from slipped discs have obtained relief by the regular practice of Dhanurāsana and Śalabhāsana (Plate 26) without being forced to rest or to undergo surgical treatment.

14. *Chaturaṅga Daṇḍāsana* One* (Plate 30)

Chatur means four. Aṅga means a limb or a part thereof. Daṇḍa means a staff. Lie flat on the floor, face down and take the weight of the body on the palms and toes, exhale and keep the body parallel to the floor, stiff as a staff. The four limbs supporting the body are the hands and feet. The pose is similar to dips in western gymnastics.

Technique

1. Lie flat on the floor, face downwards.

2. Bend the elbows and place the palms by the side of the chest. Keep the feet about a foot apart.

3. With an exhalation, raise the whole body a few inches above the floor, balancing it on the hands and the toes. (Plate 29) Keep the body stiff as a staff, parallel to the floor from head to heel and the knees taut. Stay for some time with normal breathing.

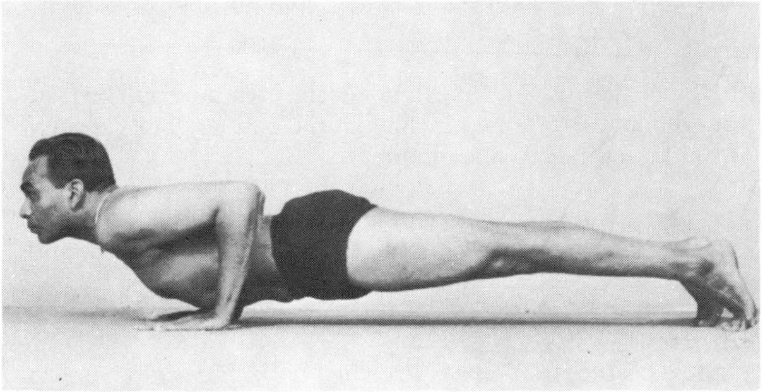

29

4. Then gradually extend the whole body forward so that the feet rest on the upper portion of the toes on the floor. (Plate 30)

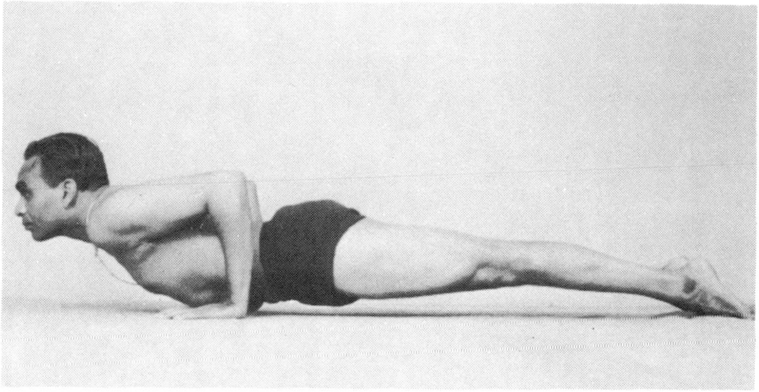

30

5. Stay in the pose for about 30 seconds with normal or deep breathing. The movement may be repeated several times. Then relax on the floor.

Effects

The pose strengthens the arms and the wrists develop mobility and power. It also contracts and tones the abdominal organs.

15. *Bhujaṅgāsana I* One* (Plate 31)

Bhujanga means a serpent. In this posture, lie flat on the floor, face downwards, lift the body up from the trunk and throw the head back like a serpent about to strike.

Technique

1. Lie on the floor face downwards. Extend the legs, keeping the feet together. Keep the knees tight and the toes pointing.

2. Rest the palms by the side of the pelvic region.

3. Inhale, press the palms firmly on the floor and lift the body up from the trunk until the pubis is in contact with the floor and stay in this position with the weight on the legs and palms. (Plate 31)

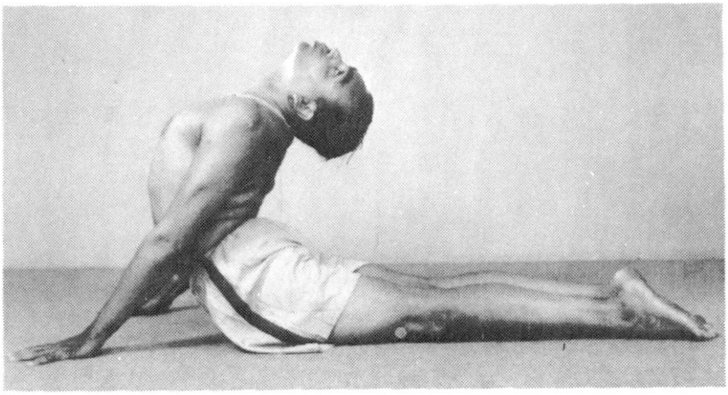

31

4. Contract the anus and the buttocks, tighten the thighs.

5. Maintain the pose for about 20 seconds, breathing normally.

6. Exhale, bend the elbows and rest the trunk on the floor. Repeat the pose two or three times and then relax.

Effects
The posture is a panacea for an injured spine and in cases of slight displacement of spinal discs the practice of this pose replaces the discs in their original position. The spinal region is toned and the chest fully expanded.

16. *Ūrdhva Mukha Śvānāsana* One* (Plate 32)
Ūrdhva Mukha means having the mouth upwards. Śvāna means a dog. The pose resembles a dog stretching itself with the head up in the air, hence the name.

Technique
1. Lie on the floor on the stomach, face downwards.

2. Keep the feet about one foot apart. The toes should point straight back. Place the palms on the floor by the side of the waist, the fingers pointing to the head.

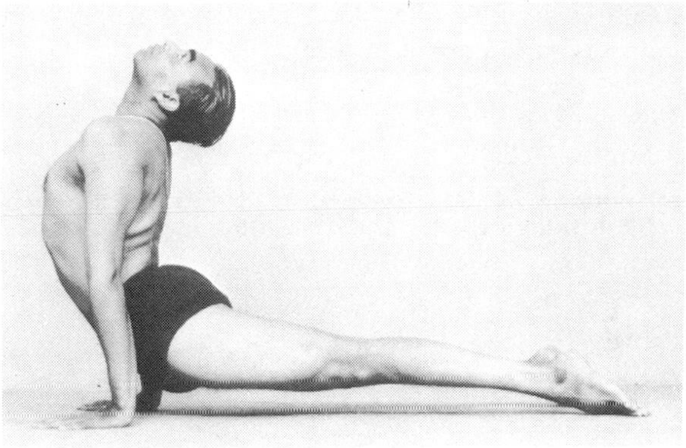

32

3. Inhale, raise the head and trunk, stretch the arms completely and push the head and trunk as far back as possible, without resting the knees on the floor.

4. Keep the legs straight and tightened at the knees, but do not rest the knees on the floor. The weight of the body rests on the palms and toes only. (Plate 32)

5. The spine, thighs and calves should be fully stretched, and the buttocks contracted tight. Push the chest forward, stretch the neck fully and throw the head as far back as possible. Stretch also the back portions of the arms.

6. Stay in the pose from half a minute to a minute with deep breathing.

7. Bend the elbows, release the stretch and rest on the floor.

Effects
The pose rejuvenates the spine and is specially recommended for people suffering from a stiff back. The movement is good for persons with lumbago, sciatica and those suffering from slipped or prolapsed discs of the spine. The pose strengthens the spine and cures backaches. Due to chest expansion, the

lungs gain elasticity. The blood circulates properly in the pelvic region and keeps it healthy.

17. *Adho Mukha Śvānāsana* Five* (Plate 33)

Adho Mukha means having the face downwards. Śvāna means a dog. The pose resembles a dog stretching itself with head and forelegs down and the hind legs up, hence the name.

Technique

1. Lie full length on the floor on the stomach, face downwards. The feet should be kept one foot apart.

2. Rest the palms by the side of the chest, the fingers straight and pointing in the direction of the head.

3. Exhale and raise the trunk from the floor. Straighten the arms, move the head inwards towards the feet and place the crown of the head on the floor, keeping the elbows straight and extending the back. (Side view: Plate 33. Back view: Plate 34)

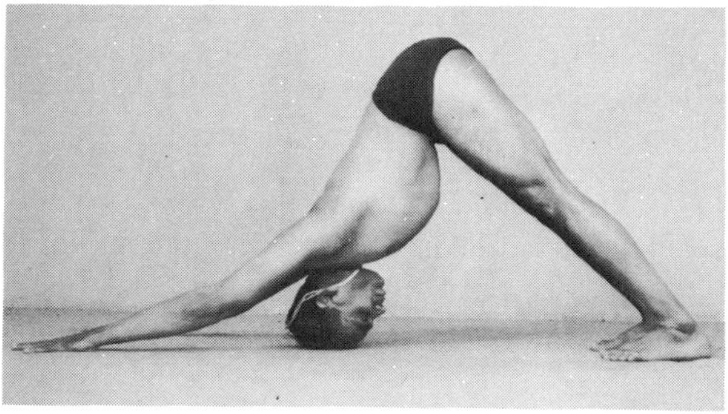

33

4. Keep the legs stiff and do not bend the knees but press the heels down. The heels and soles of the feet should rest completely on the floor, while the feet should be parallel to each other, the toes pointing straight ahead.

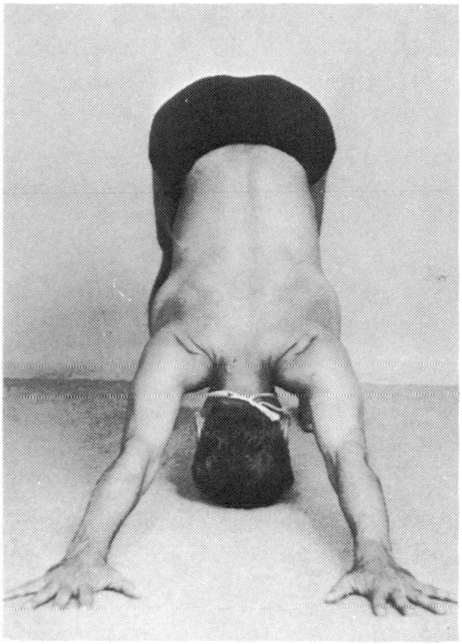

34

5. Stay in the pose for about a minute with deep breathing. Then with an exhalation lift the head off the floor, stretch the trunk forward and lower the body gently to the floor and relax.

Effects

When one is exhausted, a longer stay in this pose removes fatigue and brings back the lost energy. The pose is especially good for runners who get tired after a hard race. Sprinters will develop speed and lightness in the legs. The pose relieves pain and stiffness in the heels and helps to soften calcaneal spurs. It strengthens the ankles and makes the legs shapely. The practice of this āsana helps to eradicate stiffness in the region of the shoulder-blades, and arthritis of the shoulder joints is relieved. The abdominal muscles are drawn towards the spine and strengthened. As the diaphragm is lifted to the chest cavity the rate of the heart beat is slowed down. This is an exhilarating pose.

Those who are afraid to do Śīrṣāsana (Plate 90) can conveniently practise this position. As the trunk is lowered in this āsana it is fully stretched and healthy blood is brought to this region without any strain on the heart. It rejuvenates the brain cells and invigorates the brain by relieving fatigue.

Persons suffering from high blood pressure can do this pose.

18. *Daṇḍāsana* Two* (Plate 35)
Daṇḍa means a staff or rod.

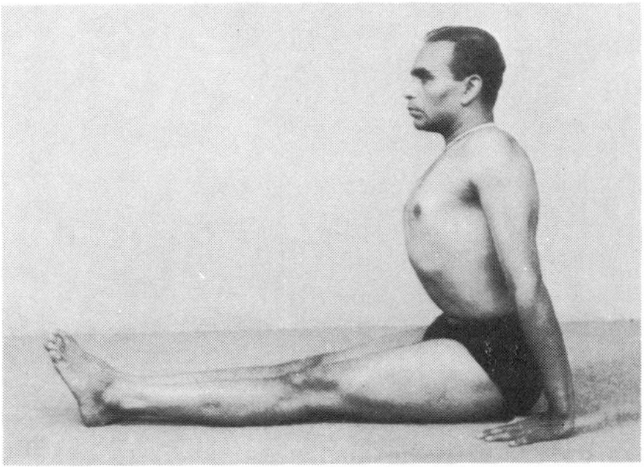

35

Technique
Sit on the floor with the legs stretched in front. Place the palms on the floor by the hips, the fingers pointing to the feet. Stretch the hands straight and keep the back erect.

19. *Paripūrṇa Nāvāsana* Two* (Plate 36)
Paripūrṇa means entire or complete. The posture here resembles that of a boat with oars, hence the name.

Technique
1. Sit on the floor as in Daṇḍāsana (18 above).

2. Exhale, recline the trunk slightly back and simultane-

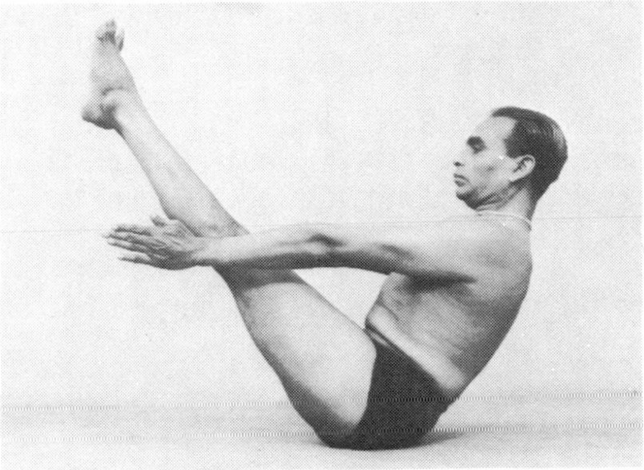

36

ously raise the legs from the floor and keep them stiff as a poker with the knees tight and the toes pointing forwards. Balance is maintained only on the buttocks and no part of the spine should be allowed to touch the floor, from which the legs should be kept at an angle of 60 to 65 degrees. The feet are higher than the head and not level with it as in Ardha Nāvāsana. (Plate 37)

3. Remove the hands from the floor and stretch the arms forward, keeping them parallel to the floor and near the thighs. The shoulders and the palms should be on one level, and the palms should face each other. (Plate 36)

4. Stay in the pose for half a minute, with normal breathing. Gradually increase the time to one minute. One feels the effect of the exercise after only 20 seconds.

5. Then exhale, lower the hands, rest the legs on the floor and relax by lying on the back.

Effects

This āsana gives relief to persons who feel a bloating sensation in the abdomen due to gas and also to those suffering from gastric complaints. It reduces fat around the waistline and tones the kidneys.

20. *Ardha Nāvāsana* Two* (Plate 37)

Ardha means half. Nāva is a ship, boat or vessel. This posture resembles the shape of a boat, hence the name.

Technique

1. Sit on the floor. Stretch the legs out in front and keep them straight. (Plate 35)

2. Interlock the fingers and place them on the back of the head just above the neck.

3. Exhale, recline the trunk back and simultaneously raise the legs from the floor, keeping the thighs and knees tight and the toes pointed. The balance of the body rests on the buttocks and no part of the spine should be allowed to touch the floor. (Plate 37.) One feels the grip on the muscles of the abdomen and the lower back.

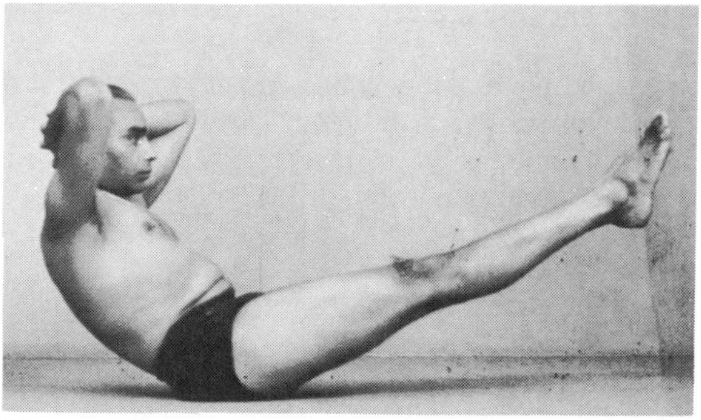

37

4. Keep the legs at an angle of about 30 to 35 degrees from the floor and the crown of the head in line with the toes.

5. Hold this pose for 20 to 30 seconds with normal breathing. A stay for one minute in this posture indicates strong abdominal muscles.

6. Do not hold the breath during this āsana, though the tendency is always to do it with suspension of breath after inhalation. If the breath is held, the effect will be felt on the stomach muscles and not on the abdominal organs. Deep inhalation in this āsana would loose the grip on the abdominal muscles. In order to maintain this grip, inhale, exhale and hold the breath and go on repeating this process but without breathing deeply. This will exercise not only the abdominal muscles but the organs also.

7. The difference between Ardha Nāvāsana and Paripūrṇa Nāvāsana should be noted; in the latter, the legs are moved higher and the distance between them and the stomach is less than in the former.

Effects

The effects of Ardha Nāvāsana and that of Paripūrṇa Nāvāsana (Plate 36) differ due to the position of the legs. In Paripūrṇa Nāvāsana the exercise is effective on the intestines; whereas, Ardha Nāvāsana works on the liver, gall bladder and spleen.

In the beginning, the back is too weak to bear the strain of the pose. When power to retain the pose comes, it indicates that the back is gaining strength. A weak back is a handicap in many ways, especially to women as they need strong backs for child-bearing. These two āsanas coupled with lateral twistings of the spine will help to strengthen the back.

The importance of having a healthy lower back can be realised if we watch old people when they sit down, get up and walk, for consciously or unconsciously they support their backs with their hands. This indicates that the back is weak and cannot withstand the strain. As long as it is strong and needs no support, one feels young though advanced in age. The two āsanas bring life and vigour to the back and enable us to grow old gracefully and comfortably.

21. *Siddhāsana* One* (Plate 38)

Siddha means a semi-divine being supposed to be of great purity and holiness, and to possess supernatural faculties called siddhis. Siddha means also an inspired sage, seer or prophet.

'The Siddhas say that as among niyamas, the most important is not to harm anyone, and among the yamas a moderate diet, so is Siddhāsana among the āsanas.'

'Of the 84 lacs of āsanas, one should always practise Siddhāsana. It purifies 72,000 nāḍīs. (Nāḍīs are channels in the human body through which nervous energy passes.)

'The yogin practising contemplation upon Ātman and observing a moderate diet, if he practises Siddhāsana for twelve years, obtains the yoga siddhis.' (Ātman means the Self and the supreme Soul. Siddhīs are supernatural faculties.)

'When Siddhāsana is mastered, the Unmanī Avasthā (Samādhi) that gives delight follows without effort and naturally.'

The soul has three avasthās or conditions which are included in a fourth. They are waking, dreaming, sleeping and what is called Turīya. 'The first condition is that of wakefulness, where the self is conscious of the common world of gross objects. It enjoys gross things. Here the dependence of body is predominant. The second condition is that of dreaming, where the self enjoys subtle things, fashioning for itself a new world of forms from the material of its waking experience. The spirit is said to roam freely unfettered by the bonds of the body. The third condition is that of sound sleep, where we have neither dreams nor desires. It is called suṣupti. In it the soul is said to become temporarily one with Brahman and to enjoy bliss. In deep sleep we are lifted above all desires and freed from the vexations of spirit. . . . The soul is divine in origin, though clogged with the flesh. In sleep it is said to be released from the shackles of the body and to regain its own nature. . . . But this (that is, the eternal dreamless sleep) is likely to be confused with sheer unconsciousness. . . . The highest is not this dreamless sleep, but another, a fourth state of the soul, a pure intuitional consciousness where there is no knowledge of objects internal or external. In deep sleep the spirit dwells in a region far above the changeful life of sense in absolute union with Brahman. The turīya condition brings out the positive aspect of the negative emphasised in the condition of deep sleep.' – Radhakrishnan in *Philosophy of the Upanishads*. This fourth condition has been thus described in the Māṇḍūkya Upanishad as follows: 'The fourth, say the wise, is not subjective experience, nor objective experience, nor experience intermediate between the two, nor is it a negative condition which is neither consciousness nor unconsciousness. It is not the knowledge of the senses, nor is it relative knowledge, nor yet inferential knowledge. Beyond the senses, beyond understanding, beyond all expression, is the fourth. It is pure unitary consciousness, wherein all awareness of the world and of multiplicity is completely obliterated. It is the supreme good. It is One without a second. It is the Self. Know it alone!'

'Rāja-Yoga, Samādhi, Unmanī, Manomanī, Immortality, Concentration, Śūnyāśūnya (void and yet non-void), Parama Pāda (the Supreme State), Amanaska (suspended operation of the mind), Advaita (non-duality), Nirālamba (without support), Nirañjana (pure), Jīvanmukti (emancipated state), Sahajāvasthā (natural state) and Turīyā (literally the Fourth), all mean the same thing. As a grain of salt thrown into water unites and becomes one with it, a like union between the Mind and the Ātman is Samādhi. When Praṇa and Manas (mind) are annihilated (absorbed), the state of harmony then arising is called Samādhi.' – *Haṭha Yoga Pradīpikā*, chapter IV, verses 3 to 6.

There is no āsana like Siddha, no kumbhaka like Kevala, no mudrā like Khecharī, and no laya (absorption of the mind) like Nāda.

(Khecharī Mudrā, literally roaming through space, is described in the *Gheraṇḍa Saṁhitā* as follows in verses 25 to 28 of the third chapter: 'Cut the lower tendon of the tongue and move the tongue constantly; rub it with fresh butter, and draw it out (to lengthen it) with an iron instrument. By practising this always, the tongue becomes long and when it reaches the space between the eyebrows, then Khecharī is accomplished. Then (the tongue being lengthened) practise turning it up and back so as to touch the palate, till at length it reaches the holes of the nostrils opening into the mouth. Close those holes with the tongue (thus stopping inspiration), and gaze on the space between the eyebrows. This is called Khecharī. By this practice there is neither fainting, nor hunger, nor thirst, nor laziness. There comes neither disease, nor decay, nor death. The body becomes divine.')

(Nāda is the inner mystical sound. Verses 79 to 101 of the fourth chapter describes it in great detail with a variety of similes. Yoga is defined as control over the aberrations of the mind. In order to control the mind it is necessary that it should first be absorbed in concentration of some object, then it is gradually withdrawn from that object and made to look within one's own self. This is where the yogi is asked to concentrate upon the inner mystical sounds. 'The mind is like a serpent, forgetting all its unsteadiness by hearing Nāda, it does not run away anywhere.' Gradually as Nāda becomes latent so does the mind along with it. 'The fire, catching the wood, is extinguished along with it (after burning it up); and so the mind also, working with Nāda, becomes latent along with it.')

Technique

1. Sit on the floor, with legs stretched straight in front. (Plate 35)

2. Bend the left leg at the knee. Hold the left foot with the hands, place the heel near the perineum and rest the sole of the left foot against the right thigh.

3. Now bend the right leg at the knee and place the right foot over the left ankle, keeping the right heel against the pubic bone.

4. Place the sole of the right foot between the thigh and the calf of the left leg.

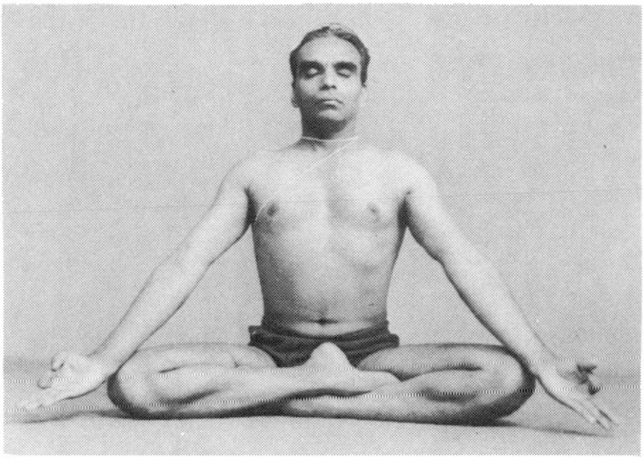

38

5. Do not rest the body on the heels.

6. Stretch the arms in front and rest the back of the hands on the knees so that the palms face upwards. Join the thumbs and the forefingers and keep the other fingers extended. (Plate 38)

7. Hold this position as long as you can, keeping the back, neck and head erect and the vision indrawn as if gazing at the tip of the nose.

8. Release the feet and relax for some time. Then repeat the pose for the same length of time, now placing the right heel near the perineum first and then the left foot over the right ankle as described above.

Effects

This posture keeps the pubic region healthy. Like Padmāsana (Plate 53), it is one of the most relaxing of āsanas. The body being in a sitting posture is at rest, while the position of the crossed legs and erect back keeps the mind attentive and alert. This āsana is also recommended for the practice of prāṇāyāma and for meditation.

From the purely physical point of view, the āsana is good for curing stiffness in the knees and ankles. In it the blood circulates in the lumbar region and the abdomen, and this tones the lower region of the spine and the abdominal organs.

22. *Vīrāsana* One* (Plates 42 and 43)
Vīra means a hero, warrior, champion. This sitting posture is done by keeping the knees together, spreading the feet and resting them by the side of the hips.

The pose is good for meditation and prāṇāyāma.

Technique

1. Kneel on the floor. Keep the knees together and spread the feet about 18 inches apart.

2. Rest the buttocks on the floor, but not the body on the feet. The feet are kept by the side of the thighs, the inner side of each calf touching the outer side of its respective thigh. Keep the toes pointing back and touching the floor. Keep the wrists on the knees, palms facing up, and join the tips of the thumbs and forefingers. Keep the other fingers extended. Stretch the back erect. (Back view: Plate 42. Front view: Plate 43)

3. Stay in this position as long as you can, with deep breathing.

4. Now interlock the fingers and stretch the arm straight over the head, palms up. (Plate 44)

5. Stay in this position for a minute with deep breathing.

6. Exhale, release the fingerlock, place the palms on the soles, bend forward and rest the chin on the knees. (Plate 45)

7. Stay in this position for a minute with normal breathing.

8. Inhale, raise the trunk up, bring the feet forward and relax.

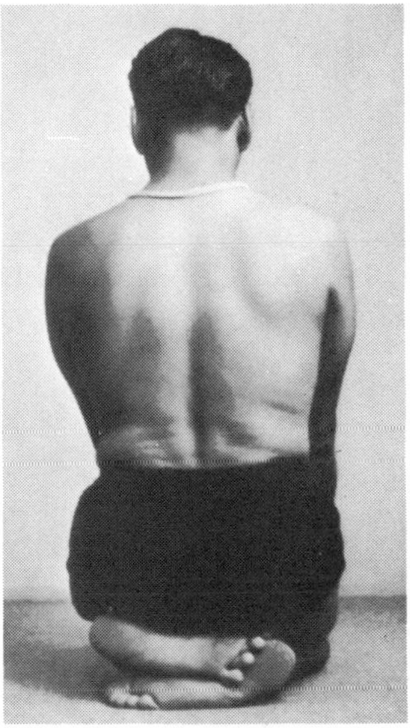

39

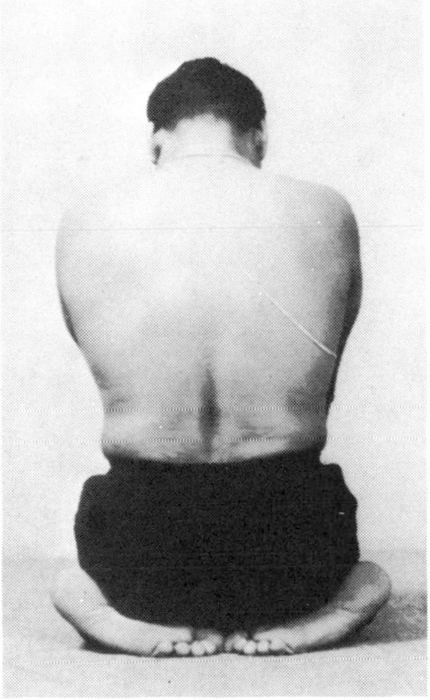

40

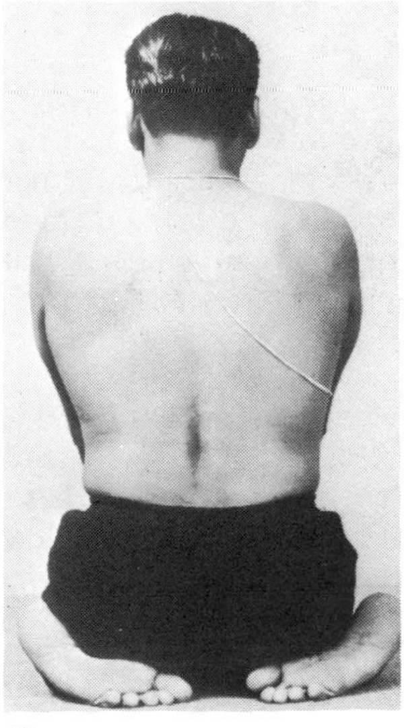

41

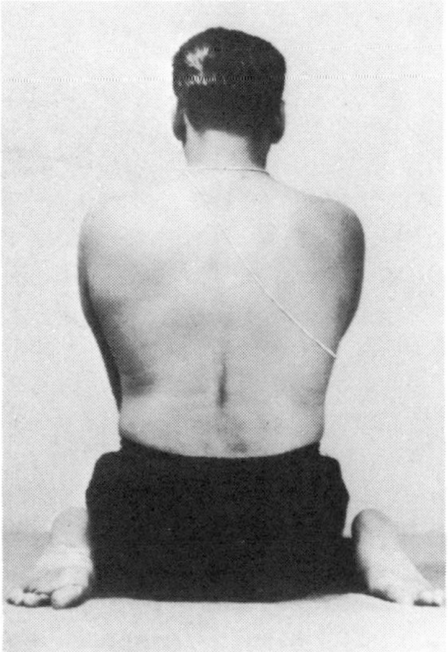

42

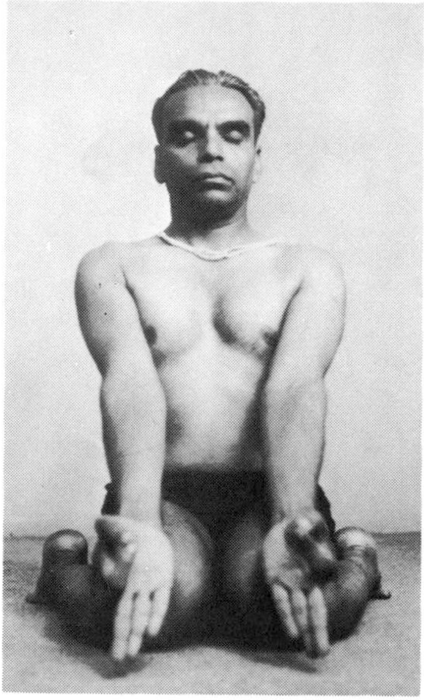

43

9. If you find it difficult to perform the pose as described above, try placing the feet one above the other and rest the buttocks on them. (Plate 39) Gradually move the toes further apart, separate the feet (Plates 40 and 41) and bring them to rest outside the thighs. Then, in time the buttocks will rest properly on the floor and the body will not rest on the feet.

Effects

The pose cures rheumatic pains in the knees and gout, and is also good for flat feet. Due to the stretching of the ankles and the feet, proper arches will be formed. This, however, takes a long time and requires daily practice of the pose for a few minutes for several months. Those suffering from pain in the heels or growth of calcaneal spurs there will get relief and the spurs will gradually disappear.

The pose can even be done immediately after food and will relieve heaviness in the stomach.

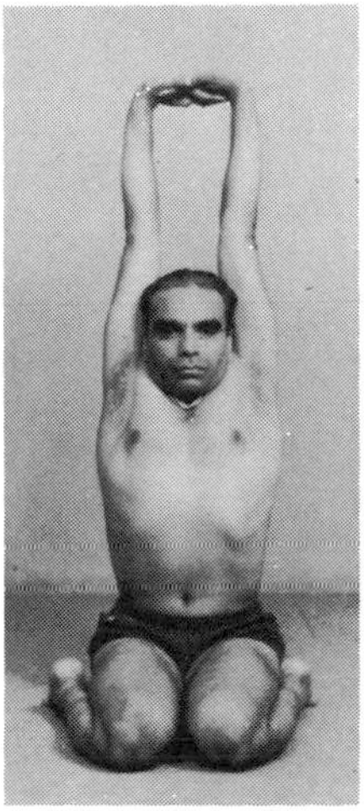

44

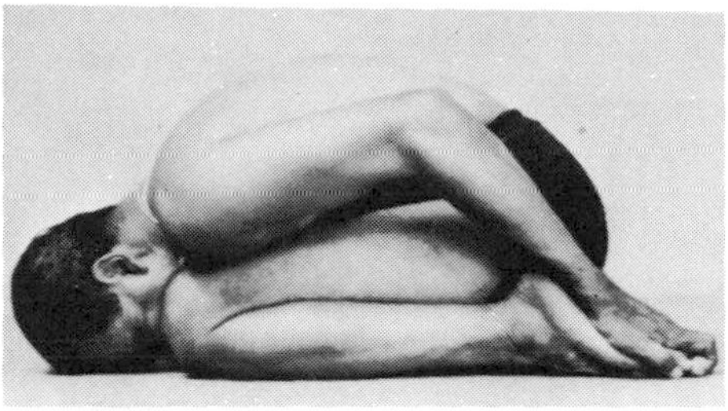

45

23. *Supta Vīrāsana* Two* (Plate 49)
Supta means lying down. In this āsana one reclines back on the floor and stretches the arms behind the head.

Technique
1. Sit in Vīrāsana. (Plate 43)

2. Exhale, recline the trunk back and rest the elbows one by one on the floor. (Plate 46)

3. Relieve the pressure on the elbows one after the other by extending the arms.

4. At first rest the crown of the head on the floor. (Plate 47) Gradually rest the back of the head and then the back on the floor. (Plate 48) Take the arms over the head and stretch them out straight. (Plate 49) Hold this pose as long as you can while breathing deeply. Then place the arms beside the trunk, press the elbows to the floor and sit up again with an exhalation.

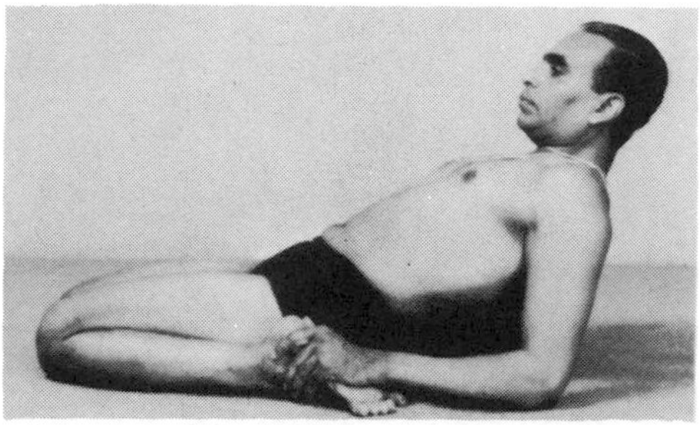

46

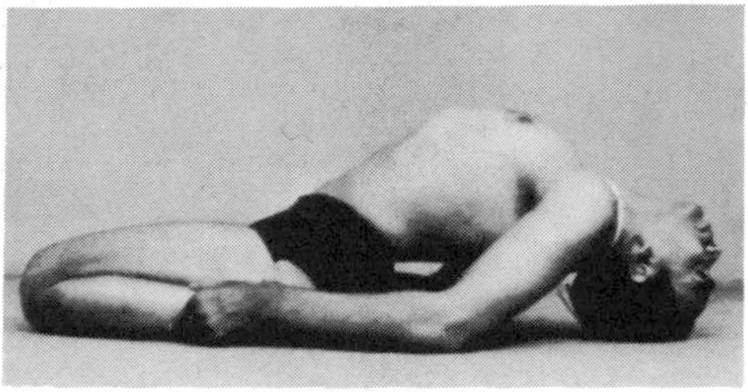

47

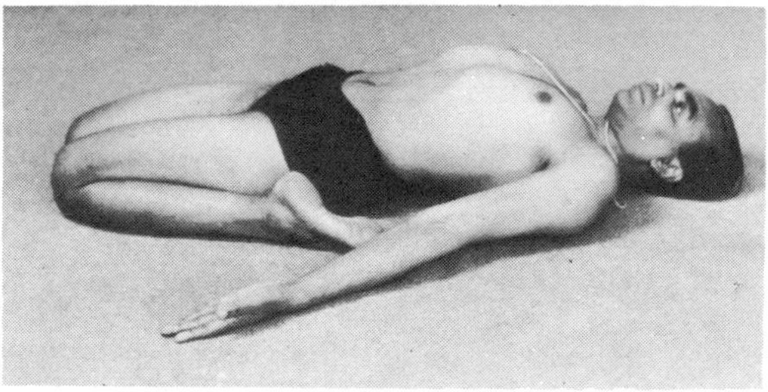

48

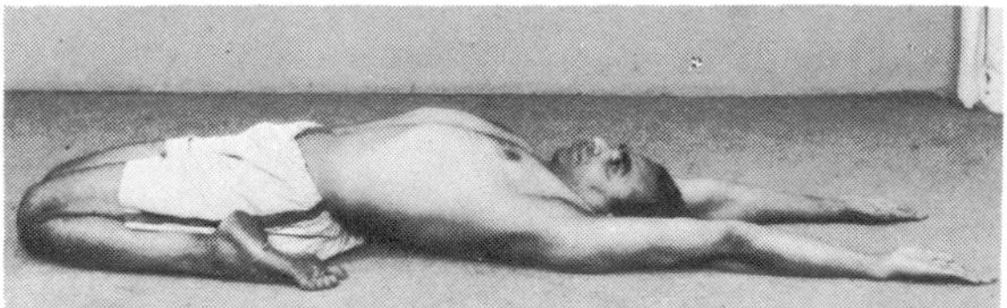

49

5. The hands may be stretched over the head or placed beside the thighs. When they are stretched over the head, do not raise the shoulder-blades from the floor.

6. Beginners may keep the knees apart.

Effects

This āsana stretches the abdominal organs and the pelvic region. People whose legs ache will get relief from holding this pose for 10 to 15 minutes and it is recommended to athletes and all who have to walk or stand about for long hours. It can be done after meals and if before retiring at night the legs feel rested next morning. Several of my pupils who were cadets at the National Defence Academy after long route marches found great relief by combining this āsana with Sarvāṅgāsana I. (Plate 102)

24. *Baddha Koṇāsana* Three* (Plate 51)

Baddha means caught, restrained. Koṇa means an angle. In this posture, sit on the floor, bring the heels near the perineum, catch the feet and widen the thighs until the knees touch the floor on either side. This is how Indian cobblers sit.

Technique

1. Sit on the floor with the legs stretched straight in front. (Plate 35)

2. Bend the knees and bring the feet closer to the trunk.

3. Bring the soles and heels of the feet together and catching the feet near the toes, bring the heels near the perineum. The outer sides of both feet should rest on the floor, and the back of the heels should touch the perineum.

4. Widen the thighs and lower the knees until they touch the floor.

5. Interlock the fingers of the hands, grip the feet firmly, stretch the spine erect and gaze straight ahead or at the tip of the nose. (Plate 50) Hold the pose as long as you can.

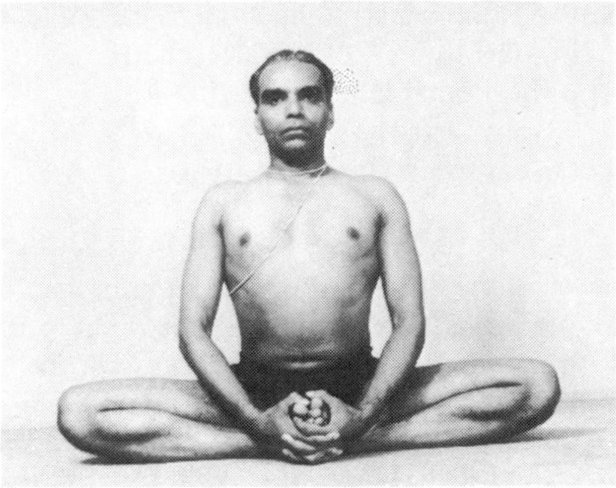

50

6. Place the elbows on the thighs and press them down. Exhale, bend forward, rest the head, then the nose and lastly the chin on the floor. (Plate 51) Hold this position from half a minute to a minute with normal breathing.

7. Inhale, raise the trunk from the floor and come back to position 5. (Plate 50)

8. Then release the feet, straighten the legs and relax.

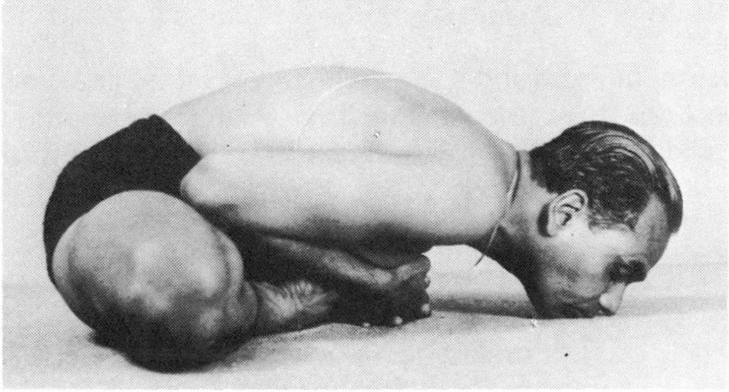

51

Effects

The pose is specially recommended for those suffering from urinary disorders. The pelvis, the abdomen and the back get a plentiful supply of blood and are stimulated. It keeps the kidneys, the prostate and the urinary bladder healthy. It is well known that diseases of the urinary tract are rarely found among the Indian cobblers and the reason for that is that they sit all day in this pose.

It relieves sciatic pain and prevents hernia. If practised regularly, it relieves pain and heaviness in the testicles.

The pose is a blessing to women. Coupled with Sarvāngāsana I (Plate 102) and its cycle (Plates 113 to 125) it checks irregular menstrual periods and helps the ovaries to function properly. It is found that pregnant women who sit daily in this pose for a few minutes will have much less pain during delivery and will be free from varicose veins. (It is recommended for pregnant women in Dr Grantly Dick Reed's book *Childbirth Without Fear*.)

Along with Padmāsana (Plate 53) and Vīrāsana (Plate 43) this āsana is recommended for Prāṇāyāma practice and for meditation. When sitting in meditation in this pose the palms should be folded in front of the chest (Plate 52), but to do this with the back erect requires practice. This āsana can be done without fear even after meals as long as the head is not rested on the floor.

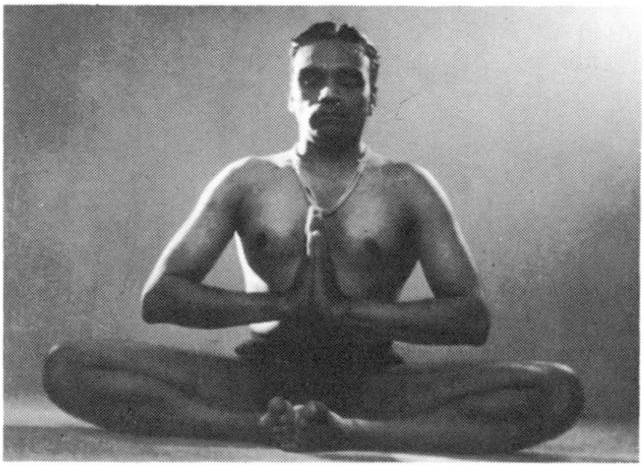

52

25. *Padmāsana* Four* (Plate 53)

Padma means a lotus. This is the lotus posture, one of the most important and useful āsanas. It is the posture for meditation and the Buddha is often depicted in it.

Verse 48 of the first chapter of the *Haṭha Yoga Pradīpikā* describes the posture and the practice of breath control while seated in it thus:

'Assuming Padmāsana and having placed the palms one upon another, fix the chin firmly upon the breast and contemplating upon Brahman, frequently contract the anus and raise the apāna up; by similar contraction of the throat force the prāna down. By this he obtains unequalled knowledge through the favour of Kuṇḍalinī (which is roused by this process).'

Kuṇḍalinī is the Divine Cosmic Energy in bodies. It is symbolised by a coiled and sleeping serpent in the lowest bodily centre at the base of the spinal column. This latent energy has to be awakened and made to go up the spine to the brain through Suṣumnā Nāḍi, a channel through which nervous energy passes, and through the six chakrās, the subtle centres in the body, the fly-wheels in the nervous system of the human machine. The awakening of Kuṇḍalinī is discussed in detail in Arthur Avalon's (Sir John Woodroffe's) book entitled *The Serpent Power*.

This is one of the basic postures and is often used in the variations of Śīrṣāsana and Sarvāngāsana.

Technique

1. Sit on the floor with the legs straight. (Plate 35)

2. Bend the right leg at the knee, hold the right foot with the hands and place it at the root of the left thigh so that the right heel is near the navel.

3. Now bend the left leg, and holding the left foot with the hands place it over the right at the root, the heel being near the navel. The soles of the feet should be turned up. This is the basic Padmāsana pose. (Plate 53)

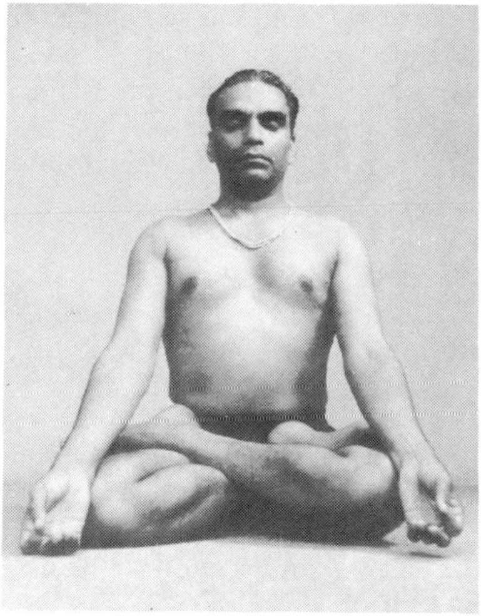

53

4. People not used to sitting on the floor seldom have flexible knees. At the start they will feel excruciating pain around the knees. By perseverance and continued practice the pain will gradually subside and they can then stay in the pose comfortably for a long time.

5. From the base to the neck the spine should remain erect. The arms may be stretched out, the right hand being placed on the right knee and the left hand on the left knee. The forefingers and the thumbs are bent and touch each other.

6. Change the leg position by placing the left foot over the right thigh and the right foot over the left thigh. This will develop the legs evenly.

Effects

After the initial knee pains have been overcome, Padmāsana is one of the most relaxing poses. The body being in a sitting posture, it is at rest without being sloppy. The position of the crossed legs and the erect back keeps the mind attentive and alert. Hence it is one of the āsanas recommended for practising prāṇāyāma (breath control).

On the purely physical level, the pose is good for curing stiffness in the knees and ankles. Since the blood is made to circulate in the lumbar region and the abdomen, the spine and the abdominal organs are toned.

26. *Parvatāsana* Four* (Plate 54)

Parvata means a mountain. In this variation of Padmāsana the arms are stretched over the head with the fingers interlocked.

Technique

1. Sit in Padmāsana. (Plate 53)

2. Interlock the fingers, and stretch the hands vertically up

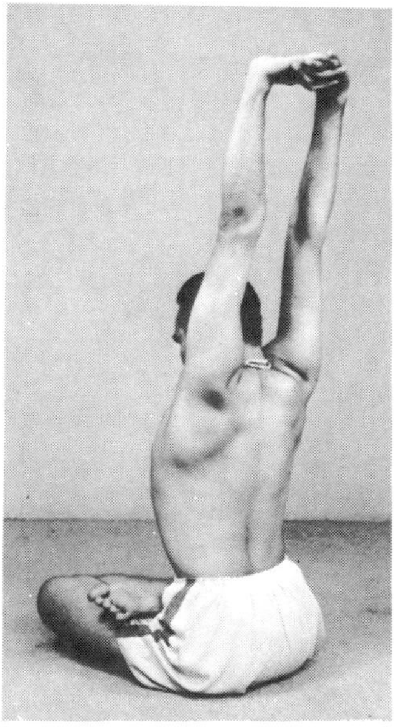

54

over the head. Keep the head bent forward with the chin on the breast bone.

3. Stretch the arms up from the latissimus dorsi (near the floating ribs at the back) and the shoulder-blades. The palms should face upwards. (Plate 54)

4. Hold the pose for a minute or two with deep and even breathing. Change the crossing of the legs and the interlock of the fingers and repeat the pose, keeping the back erect.

Effects
The āsana relieves rheumatic pains and stiffness in the shoulders. It helps draw free movement and to develop the chest. The abdominal organs are drawn in and the chest expands fully.

27. *Matsyāsana* Five* (Plate 56)
Matsya means a fish. This posture is dedicated to Matsya the Fish Incarnation of Viṣṇu, the source and maintainer of the universe and of all things. It is related that once upon a time the whole earth had become corrupt and was about to be overwhelmed by a universal flood. Viṣṇu took the form of a fish and warned Manu (the Hindu Adam) of the impending disaster. The fish then carried Manu, his family and the seven great sages in a ship, fastened to a horn on his head. It also saved the Vedas from the flood.

Technique
1. Sit in Padmāsana. (Plate 53)

2. Lie flat on the back with the legs on the floor.

3. Exhale, arch the back by lifting the neck and the chest, take the head back and rest the crown on the floor. Drag the head further back by holding the crossed legs with the hands and increase the back arch. (Plate 55)

4. Now take the hands from the legs, bend the arms, hold

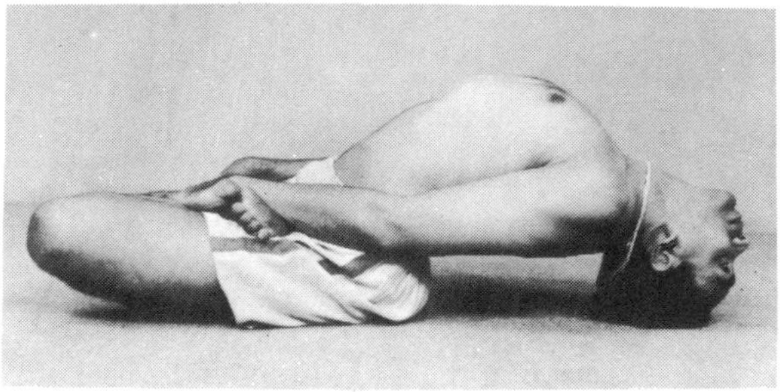

55

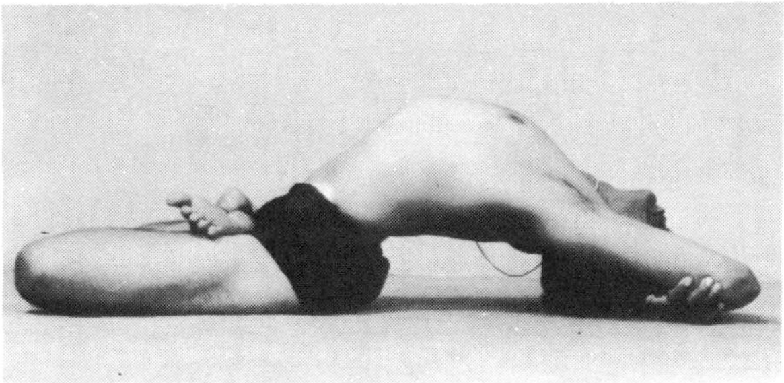

56

the elbows with the hands and rest the forearms on the floor behind the head. (Plate 56)

5. Stay in this position from 30 to 60 seconds while breathing deeply.

6. Rest the back of the head on the floor, lie flat on the back, inhale and then come up to Padmāsana, release the legs and relax.

7. Recross the legs the other way and repeat the pose for the same length of time.

8. If positions 3 and 4 are difficult to achieve, lie flat on the back with the arms stretched straight over the head. (Plate 57)

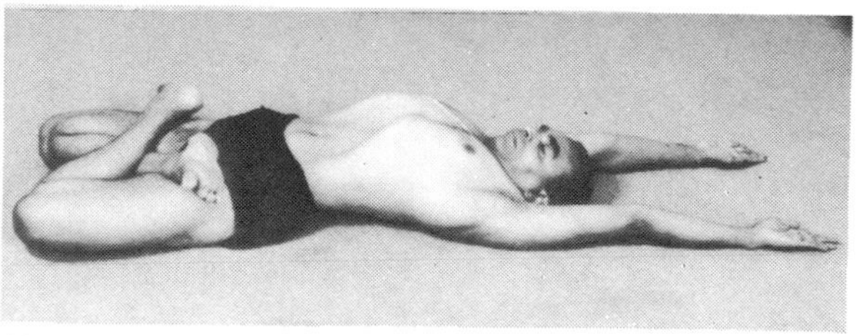

57

Effects
The dorsal region is fully extended in this posture and the chest is well expanded. Breathing becomes fuller. The thyroids benefit from the exercise due to the stretching of the neck. The pelvic joints become elastic. The āsana relives inflamed and bleeding piles.

28. *Baddha Padmāsana* Six* (Plate 58)
Baddha means caught, restrained. In this position the hands are crossed at the back and the big toes are caught from behind. The body is caught between the crossed legs in front and the crossed hands behind, hence the name.

Technique
1. Sit in Padmāsana. (Plate 53)

2. Exhale, swing the left arm back from the shoulders and bring the hand near the right hip. Catch the left big toe, hold the position and inhale.

3. Similarly, with an exhalation, swing the right arm back from the shoulder, bring it near the left hip and catch the right big toe. (Front view: Plate 58. Back view: Plate 59)

4. If the toes are difficult to catch stretch the shoulders back, so that the shoulder-blades are brought near each other. A little practice in swinging the arms back with an exhalation will enable one to catch the big toes.

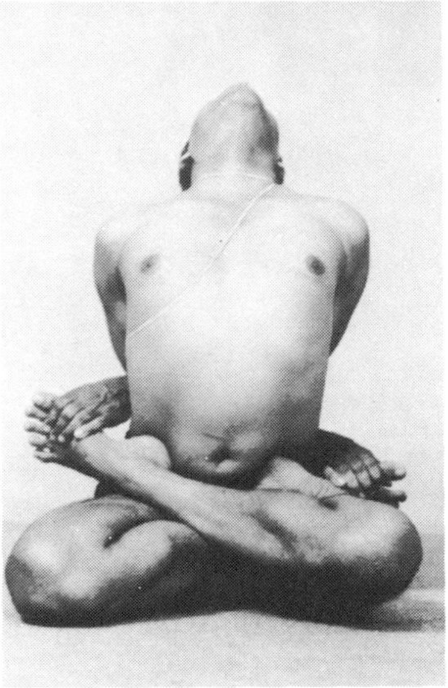

58

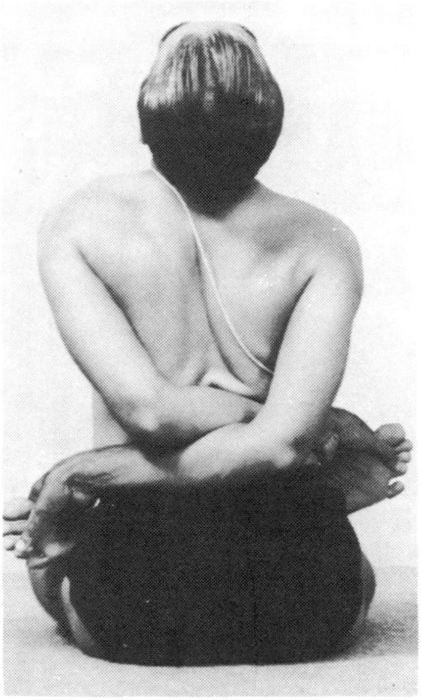

59

5. If the right foot is placed first over the left thigh and then the left foot over the right thigh, catch the left big toe first and then the right big toe. If, on the other hand, the left foot is placed over the right thigh first and then the right foot over the left thigh, catch the right big toe first and then the left big toe. Catch first the big toe of the foot which is uppermost.

6. Throw the head as far back as possible and take a few deep breaths.

7. Inhale deeply, and then with an exhalation bend the trunk forward from the hips and rest the head on the floor, without releasing the toes from the hand grip. Bending the head forward in Baddha Padmāsana (Plate 58) and touching it on the floor is called:

29. *Yoga Mudrāsana* Six* (Plate 60)
This āsana is especially useful in awakening Kuṇḍalinī.

Effects

Crossing the hands behind the back expands the chest and increases the range of shoulder movement. Yoga Mudrāsana (Plate 60) intensifies the peristaltic activity and pushes down the accumulated waste matter in the colon and thereby relieves constipation and increases digestive power.

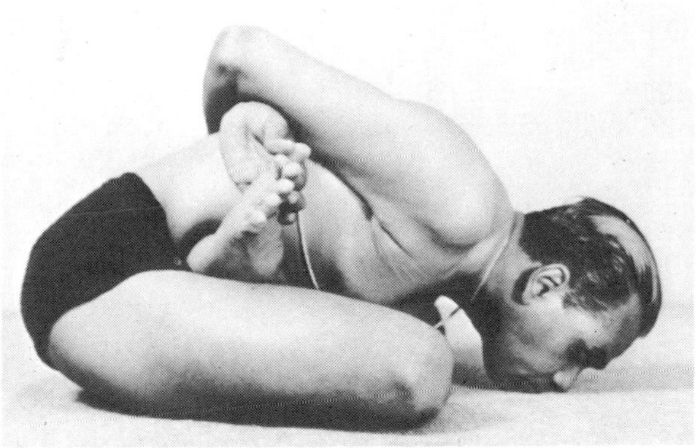

60

30. *Mahā Mudrā* Five* (Plate 61)

Mahā means great or noble. Mudrā means shutting, closing or sealing. In this sitting posture the apertures at the top and bottom of the trunk are held fast and sealed.

Technique

1. Sit on the floor with the legs stretched in front. (Plate 35)

2. Bend the left knee and move it to the left, keeping the outer side of the left thigh and the left calf on the floor.

3. Place the left heel against the inner side of the left thigh near the perineum. The big toe of the left foot should touch the inner side of the right thigh. The angle between the extended right leg and the bent left leg should be a right angle of 90 degrees.

4. Stretch the arms forward towards the right foot and hook the big toe with the thumbs and forefingers.

5. Lower the head to the trunk until the chin rests in the hollow between the collar bones just above the breast-bone.

6. Keep the spine fully stretched and do not allow the right leg to tilt to the right.

7. Inhale completely. Tighten the entire abdomen from the anus to the diaphragm. Pull the abdomen back towards the spine and also up towards the diaphragm.

8. Relax the abdominal tension, then exhale, again inhale and hold the breath, maintaining the abdominal grip. Hold this posture as stated above from one to three minutes. (Plate 61)

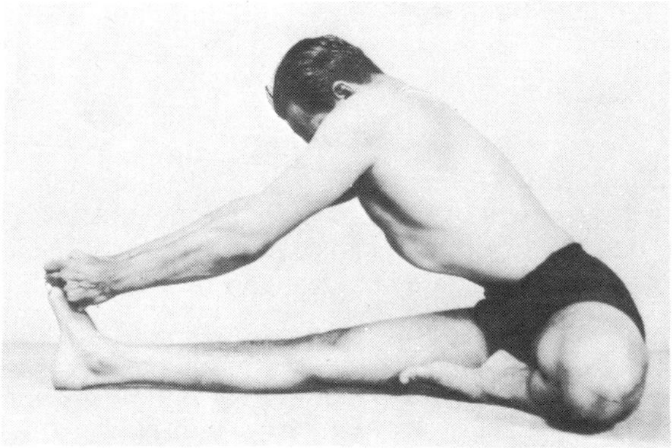

61

9. Relax the abdominal tension, exhale, raise the head, release the hands and straighten the bent leg.

10. Repeat on the other side, keeping the left leg straight and the right one bent for an equal length of time.

Effects
This āsana tones the abdominal organs, the kidneys and adrenal glands. Women suffering from a prolapsed womb find relief as it pulls the womb up to its original position. Persons suffering from spleen ailments and from enlargement of the prostate gland will benefit by staying in this pose longer. It cures indigestion.

'This Mahāmudrā destroys death and many other pains.' 'There is nothing that one cannot eat or has to avoid (if one has practised it). All food regardless of taste and even when deadly poisonous is digested.' 'He who practices Mahāmudrā, overcomes consumption, leprosy, piles, enlargement of the spleen, indigestion and other complaints of long duration.' (*Haṭha Yoga Pradīpikā,* chapter 3, verses 14, 16 and 17.)

31. *Jānu Śīrṣāsana* Five* (Plate 63)
Jānu means the knee. Śīrṣa is the head. In this posture sit with one leg stretched out on the ground and the other bent at the knee. Then catch the extended foot with both the hands and place the head on that knee.

Technique
1. Sit on the floor, with legs stretched straight in front. (Plate 35)

2. Bend the left knee and move it to the left, keeping the outer side of left thigh and the left calf on the floor.

3. Place the left heel against the inner side of the left thigh near the perineum. The big toe of the left foot should touch the inner side of the right thigh. The angle between the two legs should be obtuse. Do not keep the left knee in line with the left thigh at a right angle to the extended right leg. Try and push the left knee as far back as possible, so that the body is stretched from the bent leg.

4. Extend the arms forward towards the right foot and hold it with the hands. First catch the toes of the right foot, then

gradually catch the sole, then the heel and finally extend the arms and catch the wrist of one hand with the other, beyond the outstretched foot. (Plate 62)

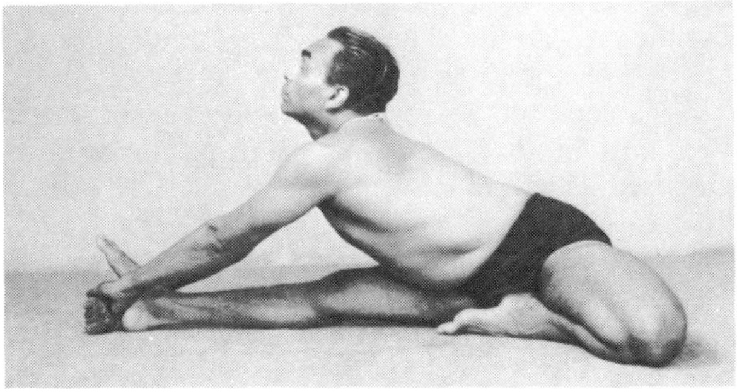

62

5. Keep the right leg stretched throughout by tightening the knee. See that the back of the right knee rests on the floor.

6. Exhale, move the trunk forward by bending and widening the elbows, and rest first the forehead, then the nose, then the lips and lastly the chin beyond the right knee. (Plate 63) The right foot will tilt to the right in the beginning. Do not allow the leg to tilt.

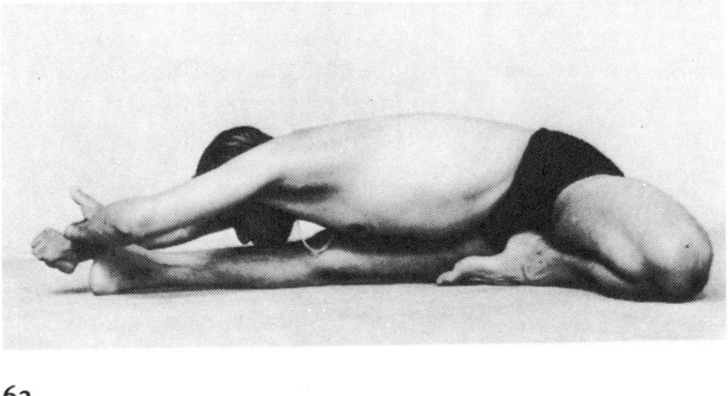

63

7. Stretch the back fully, pull the trunk forward and keep the chest against the right thigh.

8. Stay in this position with deep breathing from half a minute to a minute. One can also do the pose holding the breath after each exhalation.

9. Inhale, raise the head and trunk, straighten the arms and gaze up for a few seconds, extending the spine and trying to make it concave. (Plate 62)

10. Release the hand grip on the right foot, straighten the left leg and come back to position 1.

11. Repeat the pose keeping the left leg stretched out and bending the right leg at the knee. Stay in the pose for the same length of time on both the sides.

Effects

This āsana tones the liver and the spleen and thereby aids digestion. It also tones and activates the kidneys, the effect on which can be felt while one is performing the pose as explained above.

Persons suffering from enlargement of the prostate gland will benefit by staying longer in this pose. They should practise this āsana along with Sarvāngāsana. (Plate 102)

The pose is also recommended for people suffering from low fever for a long time.

32. *Ardha Baddha Padma Paschimottānāsana* Eight* (Plate 66)

Ardha means half, baddha means caught, restrained and padma a lotus. Paschimottānāsana (Plate 81) is the posture where the back of the whole body is intensely stretched.

Technique

1. Sit on the floor, with the legs stretched straight in front. (Plate 35)

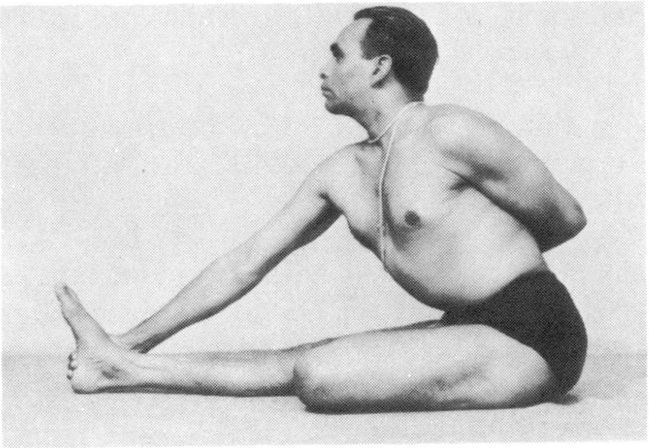

64

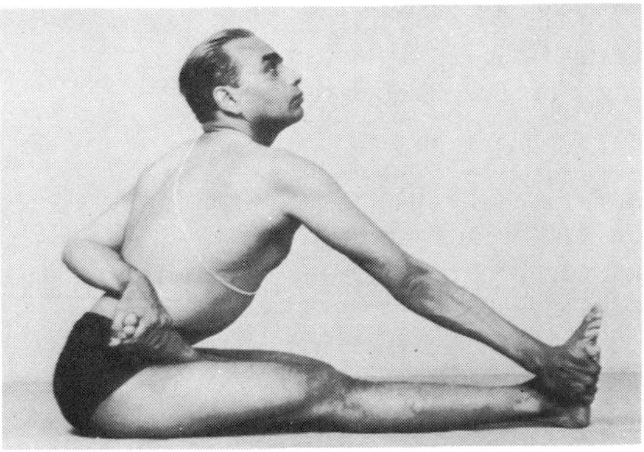

65

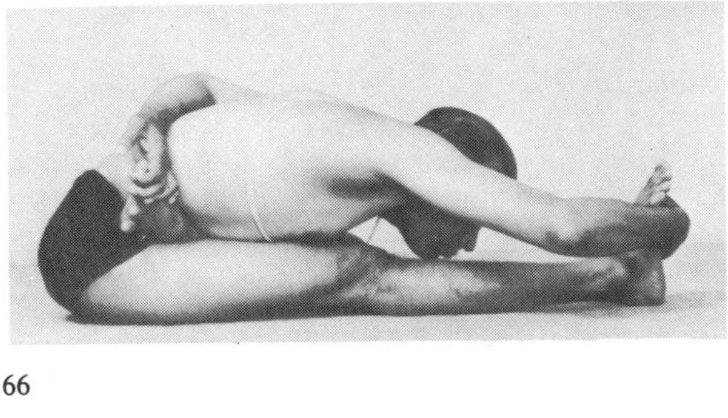

66

2. Bend the left leg at the knee, and place the left foot over the right thigh. The left heel should press the navel and the toes should be stretched and pointing. This is the half lotus posture.

3. Bring the left arm round the back from behind and with an exhalation catch the big toe of the left foot. If the toe cannot be grasped easily, swing back the left shoulder.

4. After holding the left big toe, move the bent left knee nearer to the extended right leg. Stretch the right arm forward and catch the right foot with the right hand, thc palm touching the sole. (Plates 64 and 65)

5. Inhale, stretch the back and gaze up for a few seconds, without releasing the grip on the left big toe.

6. Exhale, move the trunk forward by bending the right elbow outwards. Rest the forehead, then the nose, then the lips and lastly the chin on the right knee. (Plate 66)

7. In the initial stages, the knee of the extended leg will be lifted off the floor. Tighten the thigh muscles and rest the entire back of the extended right leg on the floor.

8. Stay in this position from 30 to 60 seconds, breathing evenly.

9. Inhale, raise the head and trunk, release the hands, straighten the left leg and come to position 1.

10. Repeat the pose on the other side, keeping the left leg stretched out on the ground, bending the right knee and placing the right foot on the left thigh. Stay for the same length of time on both sides.

11. If you cannot hold the toe with the hand from behind, hold the extended leg with both hands and follow the above techniques. (Plate 67)

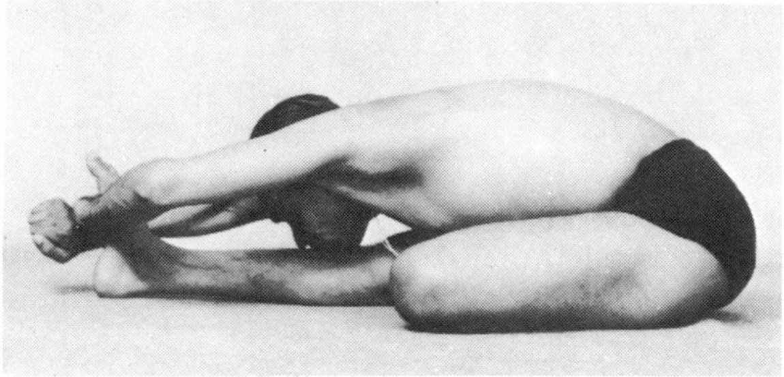

67

Effects
Due to the half lotus pose, the knees become flexible enough to execute the full lotus pose. While placing the chin on the knee of the extended leg, the bent knee is brought close to the stretched leg. This gives a good pull to the navel and abdominal organs. Blood is made to flow round the navel and the genital organs. The navel is considered to be a nerve centre, and the Svādhiṣṭhāna Chakra, one of the purificatory fly-wheels in the human nervous system, is situated there. This chakra corresponds to the hypo-gastric plexus. The pose is recommended for persons with rounded and drooping shoulders.

33. *Triaṅgā Mukhaikapda Paschimottānāsana* Five* (Plate 69)
Trianga means three limbs or parts thereof. In this posture the three parts are the feet, knees and buttocks. Mukhaikapāda (a compound of three words, mukha=face, eka=one, and pāda=leg or foot) corresponds to the face (or mouth) touching one (extended) leg. In Paschimottānāsana (Plate 81) the back of the whole body is intensely stretched.

Technique
1. Sit on the floor, with the legs stretched straight in front. (Plate 35)

2. Bend the right leg at the knee and move the right foot

back. Place the right foot by the side of the right hip joint, keep the toes pointing back and rest them on the floor. The inner side of the right calf will touch the outer side of the right thigh.

3. Balance in this position, throwing the weight of the body on the bent knee. In the beginning, the body tilts to the side of the outstretched leg, and the foot of the outstretched leg also tilts outwards. Learn to balance in this position, keeping the foot and toes stretched and pointing forward.

4. Now hold the left foot with both the palms, gripping the sides of the sole. If you can, then extend the trunk forward and hook the wrists round the outstretched left foot. (Plate 68) Take two deep breaths. It usually takes several months before one can hook the wrists in this way, so do not despair after the first few attempts.

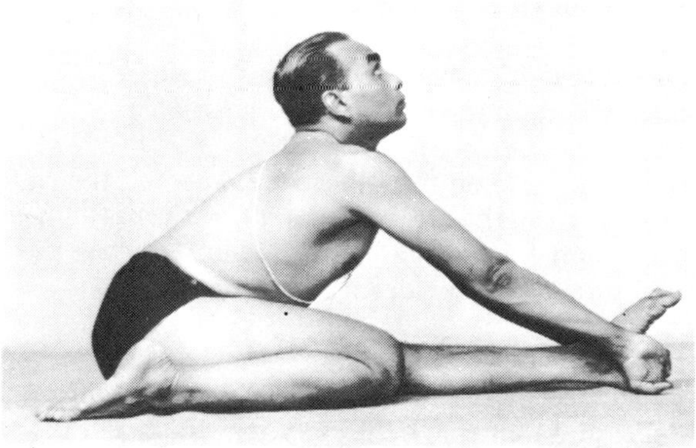

68

5. Join the knees, exhale and bend forward. Rest first the forehead, then the nose, next the lips and ultimately the chin on the left knee. (Plate 69) To achieve this, widen the elbows and push the trunk forward with an exhalation.

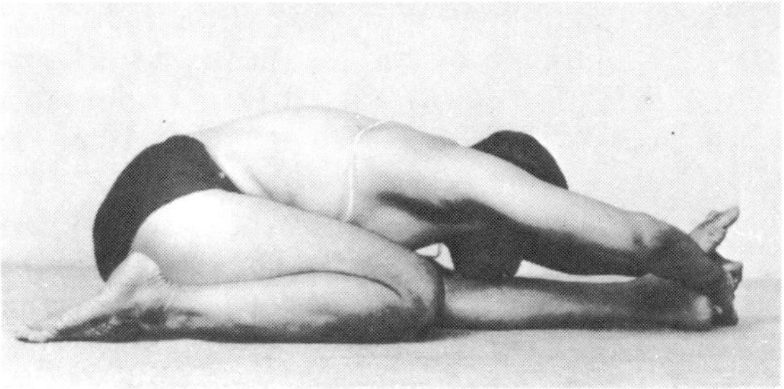

69

6. Do not rest the left elbow on the floor. In the beginning, one loses balance and topples over to the side of the extended leg. The trunk should, therefore, be slightly bent towards the side of the bent leg and the weight of the body should be taken by the bent knee.

7. Stay in this position from half a minute to a minute, breathing evenly.

8. Inhale, raise the head and trunk, release the hands, straighten the right leg and come to position 1.

9. Repeat the pose on the other side, keeping the right leg stretched out on the ground, bending the left knee and placing the left foot by the left hip joint. Stay for the same length of time on both sides.

Effects

This āsana is recommended for persons suffering from dropped arches and flat feet. It cures sprains in the ankle and the knee, and any swelling in the leg is reduced.

Along with Jānu Śīrṣāsana (Plate 63) and Ardha Baddha Padma Paschimottānāsana (Plate 66), this āsana tones the abdominal organs and keeps them free from sluggishness. We abuse our abdominal organs by over-indulgence or by conforming to social etiquette. Abdominal organs cause a majority of diseases and ancient sages emphasised that their health was essential for longevity, happiness and peace of mind. These forward bending āsanas keep the abdominal organs healthy and in trim. Apart from keeping the muscles in shape, they work on the organs as well.

34. *Marīchyāsana I* Five* (Plate 71)
This āsana is dedicated to the sage Marīchi, son of the Creator, Brahmā. Marīchi was the grandfather of Sūrya (the Sun God).

Technique

1. Sit on the floor with the legs stretched straight in front. (Plate 35)

2. Bend the left knee and place the sole and heel of the left foot flat on the floor. The shin of the left leg should be perpendicular to the floor and the calf should touch the thigh. Place the left heel near the perineum. The inner side of the left foot should touch the inner side of the outstretched right thigh.

3. Stretch the left shoulder forward till the left armpit touches the perpendicular left shin. Turn the left arm round the left shin and thigh, bend the left elbow and throw the left forearm behind the back at the level of the waist. Then move the right hand behind the back and clasp the left hand with the right at the wrist or vice versa. If that is not possible then clasp the palms or the fingers. (Plate 70)

4. Now, turn the spine to the left, keeping the outstretched right leg straight. Remain in this position gazing at the outstretched right big toe and take a few deep breaths.

5. Exhale, and bend forward. Rest the forehead, then the nose, next the lips and lastly the chin on the right knee. (Plate 71) While in this position, keep both shoulders parallel to the floor and breathe normally. Stay in the pose for about 30 seconds and see that the back of the entire extended leg rests on the floor throughout.

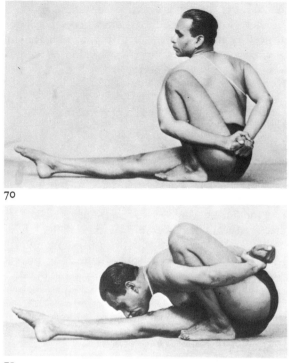

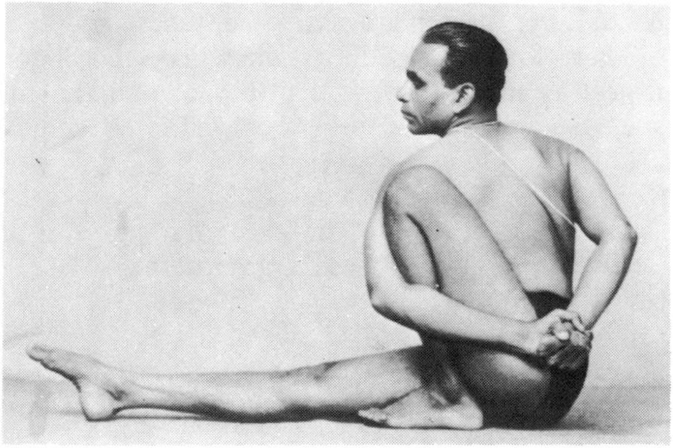

70

71

6. Inhale, raise the head from the right knee (Plate 70), release the hands, straighten the left leg and come to position 1.

7. Repeat the pose on the other side for an equal length of time.

Effects

The fingers gain in strength by the practice of this āsana. In the preceding āsanas (namely, Jānu Śīrṣāsana (Plate 63), Ardha Baddha Padma Paschimottānāsana (Plate 66) and

Triang Mukhaikapāda Paschimottānāsana (Plate 69) the abdominal organs are made to contract by gripping a leg with the hands. In this pose the hands do not hold the legs. To bend forward and to rest the chin on the knee of the extended leg the abdominal organs have to contract vigorously. This creates a better circulation of blood round the abdominal organs and keeps them healthy. In the beginning it is very difficult to bend forward at all after gripping both hands behind the back, but it comes with practice. The dorsal region of the spine is also exercised in this pose.

Note. The four poses, Jānu Śīrṣāsana, Ardha Baddha Padma Paschimottānāsana, Triang Mukhaikapāda Paschimottānāsana and Marīchyāsana I, are preparatory poses for the correct Paschimottānāsana. (Plate 81) It is difficult for many to get a good grip on the feet in Paschimottānāsana even after several attempts. These four āsanas give one sufficient elasticity in the back and legs so that one gradually achieves the correct Paschimottānāsana (Plate 81) as described later. Once this is done with ease, these four āsanas can be practised once or twice a week instead of daily.

35. *Upaviṣṭha Koṇāsana* Nine* (Plate 74)

Upaviṣṭha means seated. Koṇa means an angle.

Technique

1. Sit on the floor with the legs stretched straight in front. (Plate 35)

2. Move the legs sideways one by one and widen the distance between them as far as you can. Keep the legs extended throughout and see that the back of the entire legs rests on the floor.

3. Catch the big toes between the respective thumbs and index and middle fingers.

4. Keep the spine erect and extend the ribs. Pull the diaphragm up and hold the pose for a few seconds with deep breaths. (Plate 72)

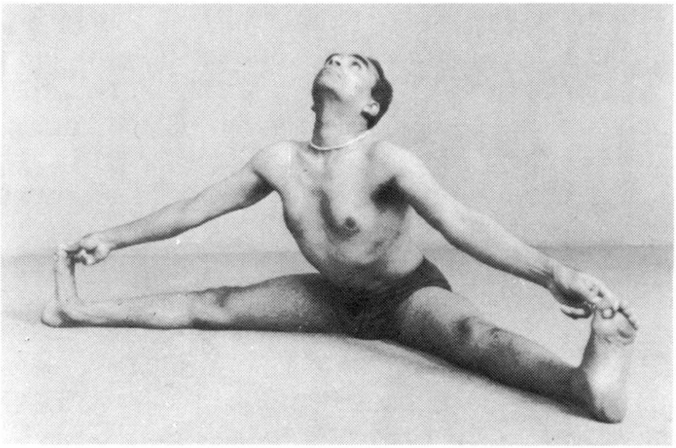

72

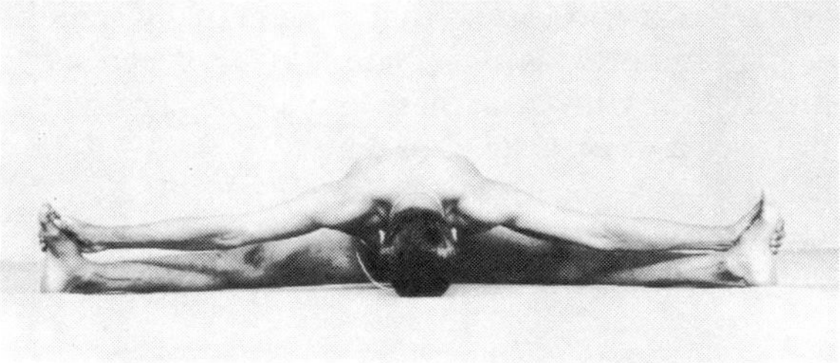

73

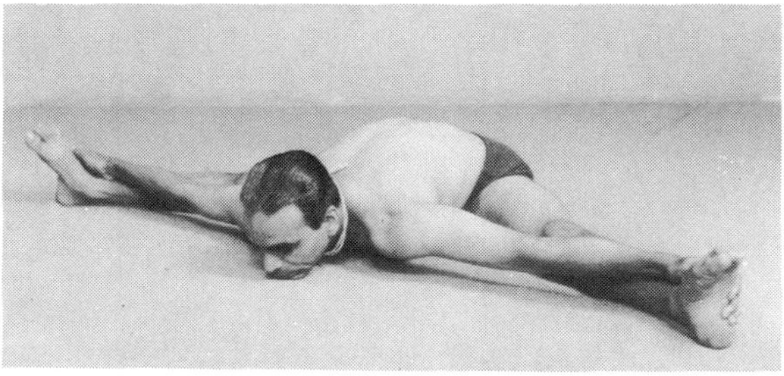

74

5. Now clasp the feet with the hands. Exhale, bend forward and rest the head on the floor. (Plate 73) Then extend the neck and place the chin on the floor.

6. Then, try to rest the chest on the floor. (Plate 74) Stay in this position from 30 to 60 seconds with normal breathing.

7. Inhale, raise the trunk off the floor (Plate 72) and release the hold on the feet, bring them together and relax.

Effects

The āsana stretches the hamstrings and helps the blood to circulate properly in the pelvic region and keeps it healthy. It prevents the development of hernia of which it can cure mild cases and relieves sciatic pains. Since the āsana controls and regularises the menstrual flow and also stimulates the ovaries, it is a boon to women.

36. *Paschimottānāsana* Six* (Plate 81)
(Also called Ugrāsana or Brahmacharyāsana)

Paschima literally means the west. It implies the back of the whole body from the head to the heels. The anterior or eastern aspect is the front of the body from the face down to the toes. The crown of the head is the upper or northern aspect while the soles and heels of the feet form the lower or southern aspect of the body. In this āsana the back of the whole body is intensely stretched, hence the name.

Ugra means formidable, powerful and noble. Brahmacharya means religious study, self-restraint and celibacy.

Technique

1. Sit on the floor with the legs stretched straight in front. Place the palms on the floor by the side of the hips. Take a few deep breaths. (Plate 35)

2. Exhale, extend the hands and catch the toes. Hold the right big toe between the right thumb and the index and middle fingers and likewise the left big toe. (Plate 75)

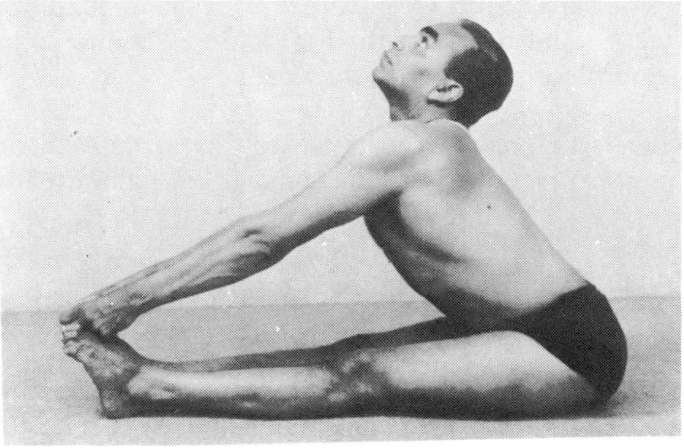

75

3. Extend the spine and try to keep the back concave. To start with the back will be like a hump. This is due to stretching the spine only from the area of the shoulders. Learn to bend right from the pelvic region of the back and also to extend the arms from the shoulders. Then the hump will disappear and the back will become flat as in Plate 75. Take a few deep breaths.

4. Now exhale, bend and widen the elbows, using them as levers, pull the trunk forward and touch the forehead to the knees. (Plate 76) Gradually rest the elbows on the floor, stretch the neck and trunk, touch the knees with the nose and then with the lips. (Plate 77)

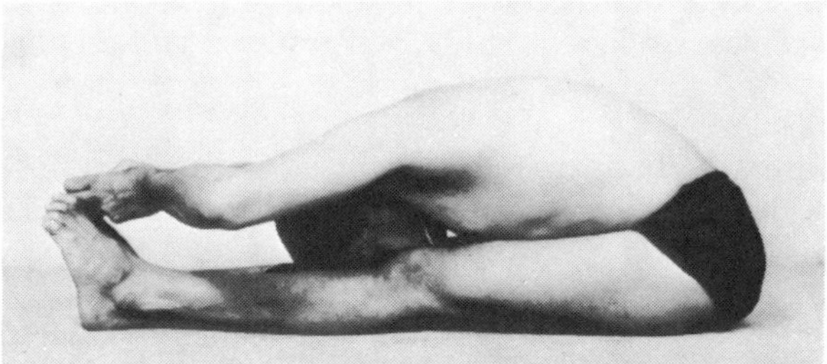

76

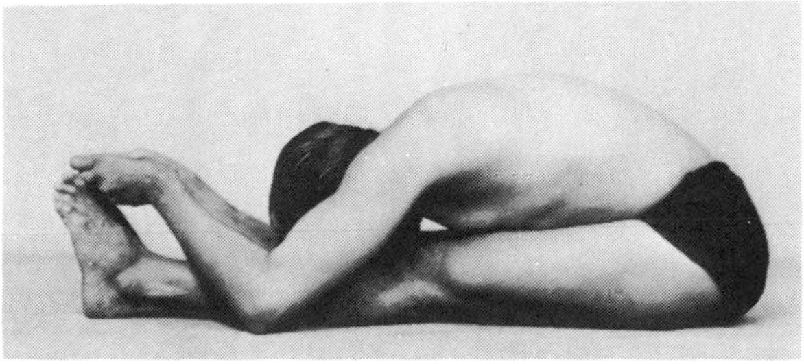

77

5. When this becomes easy, make a further effort to grip the soles and rest the chin on the knees. (Plate 78)

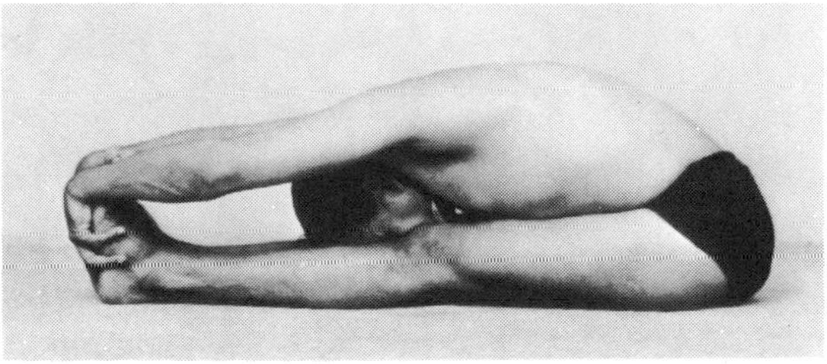

78

6. When this also becomes easy, clasp the hands by interlocking the fingers and rest the chin on the shins beyond the knees. (Plate 79)

7. When position 6 becomes easy, grip the right palm with the left hand or the left palm with the right hand beyond the outstretched feet exhale and rest the chin on the shins beyond the knees. (Plate 80)

8. If position 8 also becomes easy, hold the right wrist with the left hand or the left wrist with the right hand and rest the chin on the shins beyond the knees. (Plate 81)

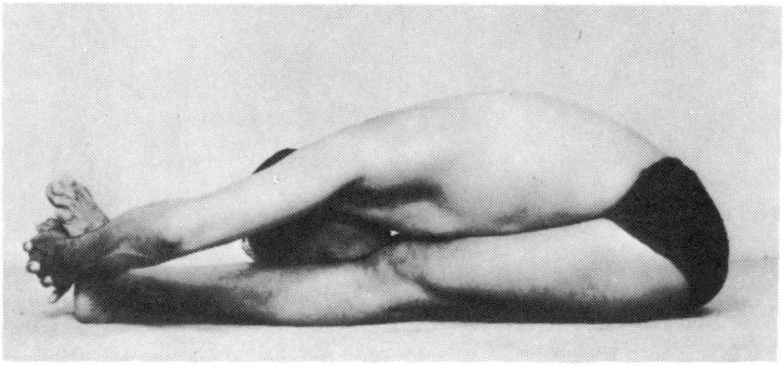

79

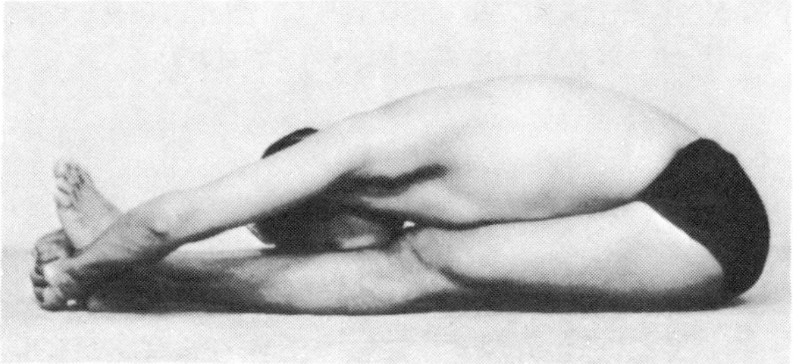

80

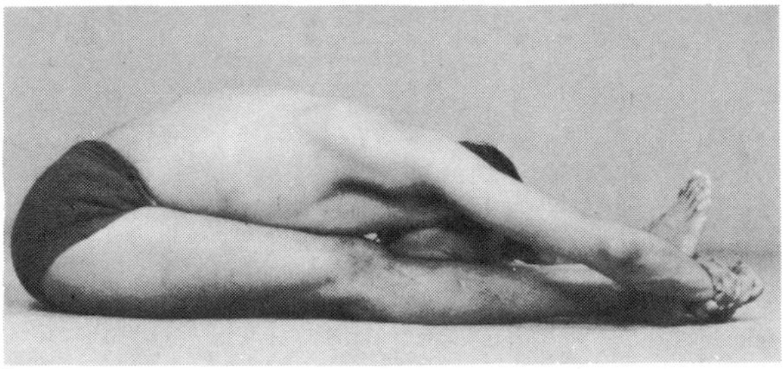

81

9. See that the back of the legs at the knee joints rests firmly on the ground. In the initial stages the knees will be lifted off the floor. Tighten the muscles at the back of the thighs and

pull the trunk forward. Then the back of the knee joints will rest on the floor.

10. Try and stay in whichever of the above positions you can achieve from 1 to 5 minutes, breathing evenly.

11. Inhale, raise the head from the knees and relax.

Effects
This āsana tones the abdominal organs and keeps them free from sluggishness. It also tones the kidneys, rejuvenates the whole spine and improves the digestion.

The spines of animals are horizontal and their hearts are below the spine. This keeps them healthy and gives them great power of endurance. In humans the spine is vertical and the heart is not lower than the spine, so that they soon feel the effects of exertion and are also susceptible to the heart diseases. In Paschimottānāsana the spine is kept straight and horizontal and the heart is at a lower level than the spine. A good stay in this pose massages the heart, the spinal column and the abdominal organs, which feel refreshed and the mind is rested. Due to the extra stretch given to the pelvic region more oxygenated blood is brought there and the gonad glands absorb the required nutrition from the blood. This increases vitality, helps to cure impotency and leads to sex control. Hence, this āsana was called Brahmacharyāsana. Brahmacharya means celibacy and a Brahmachāri is one who has controlled the sex appetite.

37. *Pūrvottānāsana* One* (Plate 82)
Pūrva literally means the East. It means the front of the whole body from the forehead to the toes. Uttāna means an intense stretch. In this posture, the whole front of the body is stretched intensely.

Technique
1. Sit on the floor with the legs stretched straight in front. Place the palms on the floor by the hips, with the fingers pointing in the direction of the feet. (Plate 35)

2. Bend the knees and place the soles and heels on the floor.

3. Take the pressure of the body on the hands and feet, exhale and lift the body off the floor. Straighten the arms and the legs and keep the knees and elbows tightened. (Plate 82)

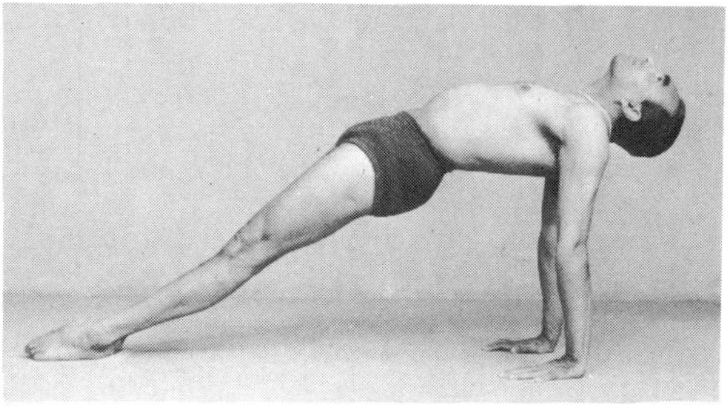

82

4. The arms will be perpendicular to the floor from the wrists to the shoulders. From the shoulders to the pelvis, the trunk will be parallel to the floor.

5. Stretch the neck and throw the head as far back as possible.

6. Stay in this posture for one minute, breathing normally.

7. Exhale, bend the elbows and knees, lower the body to sit on the floor and relax.

Effects

This posture strengthens the wrists and ankles, improves the movement of the shoulder joints and expands the chest fully. It gives relief from the fatigue caused by doing other strenuous forward bending āsanas.

38. *Sālamba Śīrṣāsana I* Four* (Plates 90, 91 and 96)

Sālamba means with support. Śīrṣa means the head. This is

the head stand pose, one of the most important Yogic āsanas. It is the basic posture. It has several variations, which are described later as the Śīrṣāsana cycle. Its mastery gives one balance and poise, both physically and mentally. The technique of doing it is given at length in two parts; the first is for beginners, the second for those who can remain balanced in the pose. Attention is specially directed to the hints on Śīrṣāsana given after the two techniques.

Technique for beginners

1. Spread a blanket fourfold on the floor and kneel near it.

2. Rest the forearms on the centre of the blanket. While doing so take care that the distance between the elbows on the floor is not wider than the shoulders.

3. Interlock the fingers right up to the finger-tips (Plate 83), so that the palms form a cup. Place the sides of the palms near the little fingers on the blankets. While going up on to your head or balancing, the fingers should be kept tightly locked. If they are left loose, the weight of the body falls on them and the arms ache. So remember to lock them well.

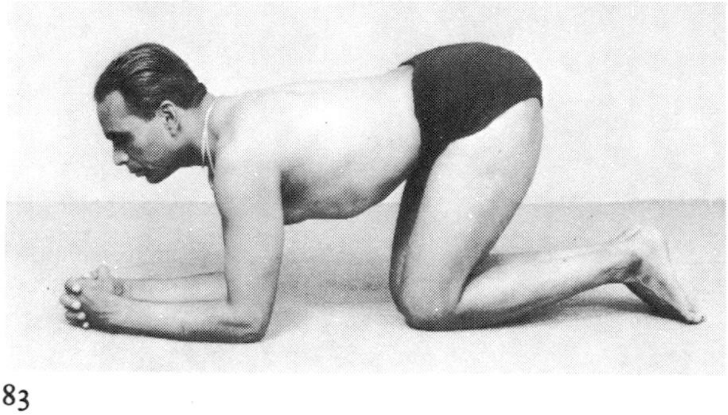

83

4. Rest the crown of the head only on the blanket, so that the back of the head touches the palms which are cupped. (Plate 84) Do not rest the forehead nor the back but only the crown

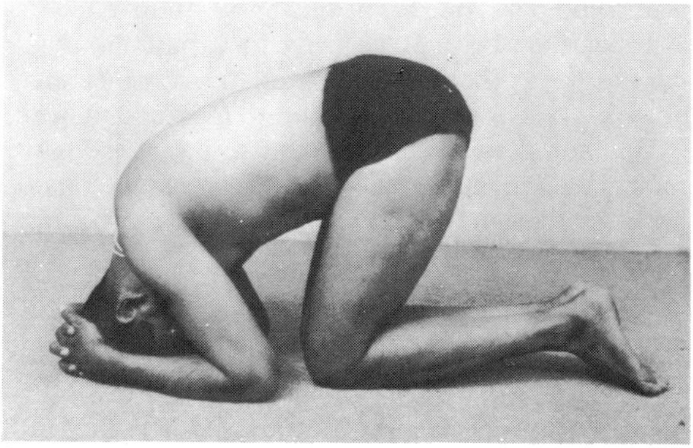

84

of the head on the blanket. To do this move the knees towards the head.

5. After securing the head position, raise the knees from the floor by moving the toes closer to the head. (Plate 85)

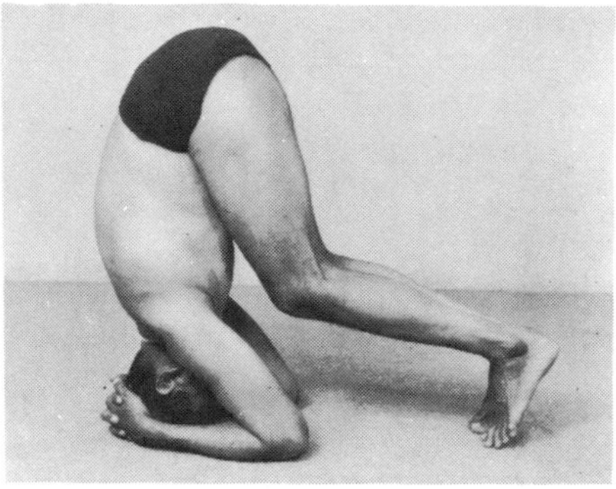

85

6. Exhale, take a gentle swing from the floor and lift the legs off the ground with bent knees. Take the swing in such a way that both feet leave the floor simultaneously, to come to position as in Plate 86. When once this position is secured,

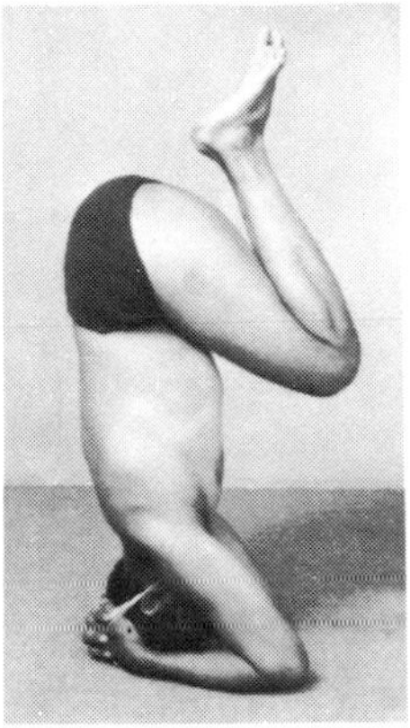

86

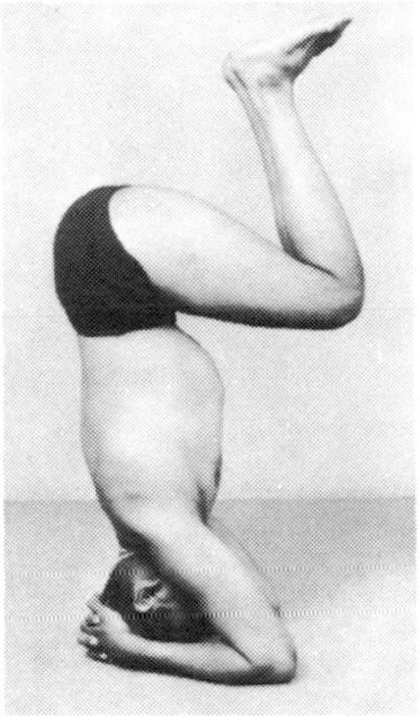

87

follow the various stages of the leg movements as in Plates 87, 88 and 89, step by step.

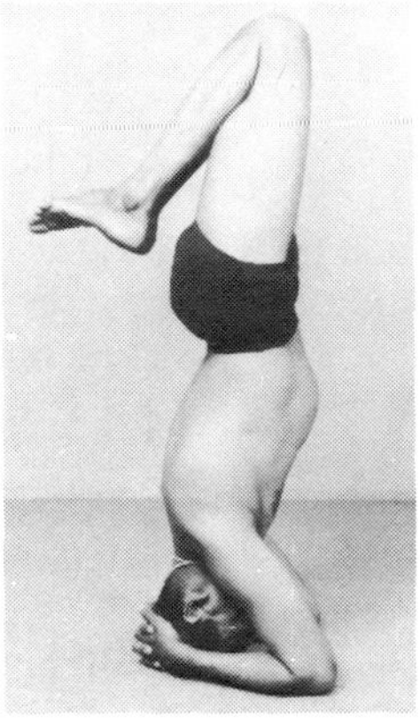

88

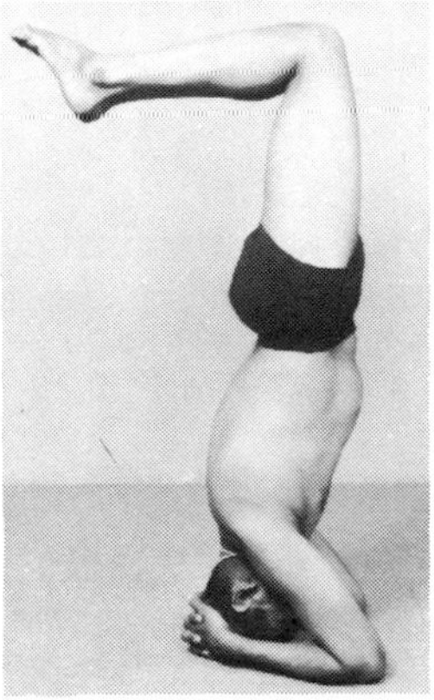

89

7. Stretch the legs and stand on the head, keeping the whole body perpendicular to the floor. (Front view: Plate 90. Back view: Plate 91. Side view: Plate 96)

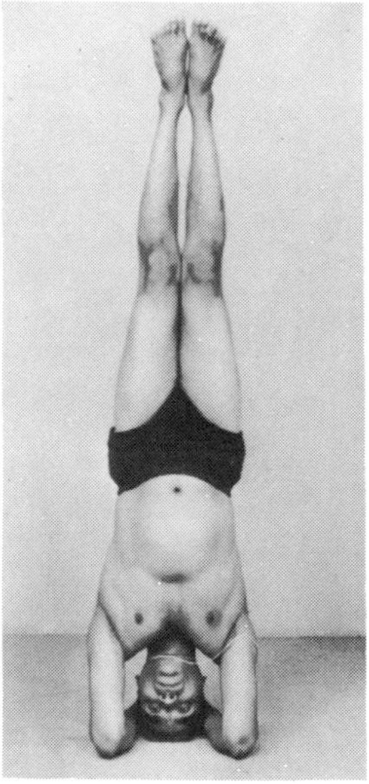

90

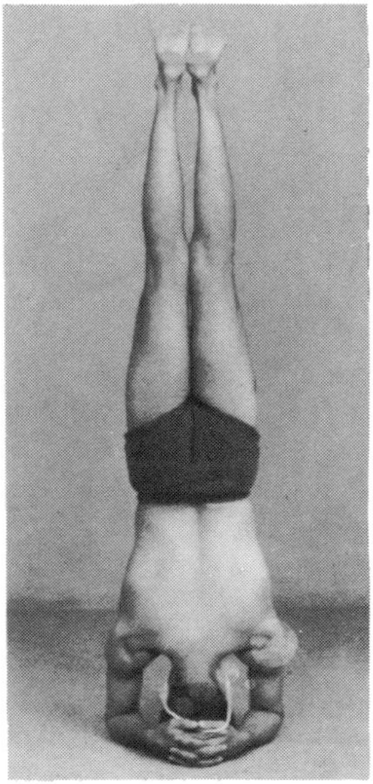

91

8. After staying in the final position to capacity, from one to five minutes, flex the knees and slide down to the floor in the reverse order as in Plates 89, 88, 87, 86, 85, 84 and raise head from the floor.

9. A beginner must have the assistance of a friend or do the āsana against a wall. While practising against a wall, the distance between it and the head should not be more than 2 or 3 inches. If the distance is greater, the spine will curve and the stomach will protrude. The weight of the body will be felt on the elbows and the position of the head may change. The face will appear to be flushed and the eyes either strained or puffed. It is, therefore, advisable for a beginner to do the head stand in a corner where two walls meet, placing the head some 2 to 3 inches from either wall.

10. While doing the head stand against a wall or in a corner, the beginner should exhale, swing the legs up, support the hips against the side of the wall and move the feet up. In a corner, he can touch the heels to either side of the walls. He should then stretch the back vertically up, gradually leave the support of the wall and learn to master the balance. While coming down, he can rest the feet and hips against the wall, slide down and kneel, resting his knees on the floor. The movements of coming down and going up should be done with an exhalation.

11. The advantage which the beginner has of balancing in a corner is that his head and legs will be in the right angle formed by the walls, and he will be sure of his right position. This will not be the case if he balances against a straight wall. For while his balance is insecure he may sway from the wall, or his body may tilt or swing to the stronger side, while his legs may rest against the wall with a bend either at the waist or the hips. The beginner will not be in a position to know that he has tilted to one side, much less to correct it. In time he may learn to balance on the head, but by habit his body may still tilt or his head may not be straight. It is as hard to correct a wrong pose in the head stand as it is to break a bad habit. Moreover this wrong posture may well lead to aches and pains in the head, neck, shoulders and back. But the two walls of a corner will help the beginner to keep the āsana symmetrical.

12. When once balance is secured, it is advisable to come down to the floor with the legs straight (that is, without bending the knees at all) and with a backward action of the hips. At first, it is not possible to go up and come down without bending the legs, but the correct method should be learnt. Once the beginner has confidence in the head stand, he will find it more beneficial to go up and down with the legs together and straight, without any jerks.

13. It takes time for the beginner to become oriented to his surroundings while he is balancing on his head. Everything

will seem at first to be completely unfamiliar. The directions and instructions will appear confusing and he will find it an effort to think clearly or to act logically. This is due to fear of a fall. The best way to overcome fear is to face with equanimity the situation of which one is afraid. Then one gets the correct perspective, and one is not frightened any more. To topple over while learning the head stand is not as terrible as we imagine. If one overbalances, one should remember to loosen the interlocked fingers, relax, go limp and flex the knees. Then one will just roll over and smile. If the fingers are not loosened they will take the jerk of the fall which will be painful. If we do not relax and go limp while falling we hit the floor with a hard bump. If we flex the knees, we are unlikely to graze them in the fall. After one has learnt to balance against a wall or in a corner, one should try the head stand in the middle of the room. There will be a few spills and one must learn the art of falling as indicated above. Learning to do Śīrṣāsana in the middle of a room gives the beginner great confidence.

Technique for those who can balance Eight*

1. Follow the technique described for beginners from positions 1 to 4.

2. After securing the head position, stretch the legs straight by raising the knees from the floor. Move the toes nearer to the head and try to press the heels to the floor, keeping the back erect. (Plate 92)

3. Stretch the dorsal or middle region of the spine and stay in this position for about 30 seconds while breathing evenly.

4. Exhale, raise the heels and take the toes off the floor with a backward movement of the hips. Raise both legs simultaneously, keeping them poker stiff. (Plate 93) Take a breath.

5. Again with an exhalation move the legs up until they are parallel to the floor. This position is called:

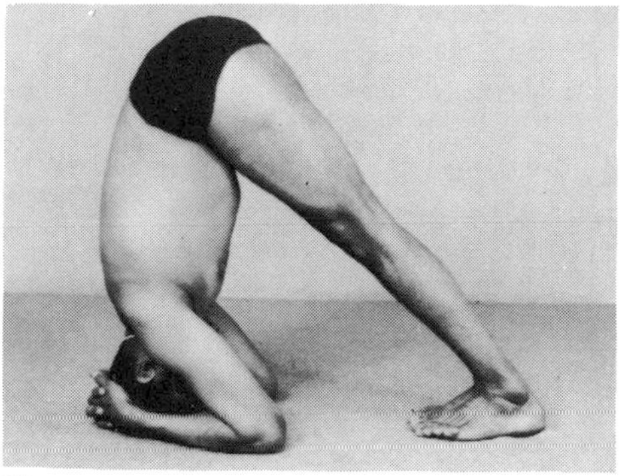

92

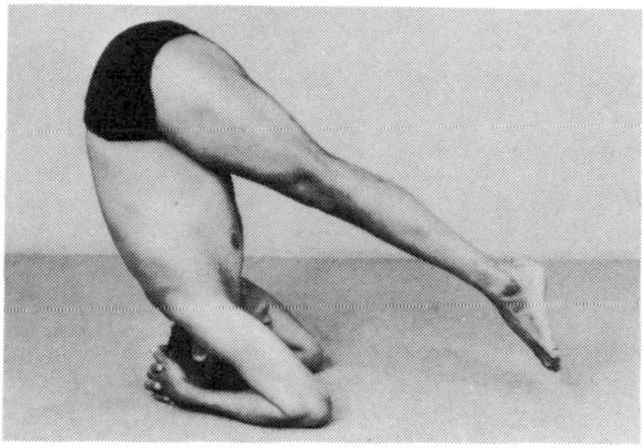

93

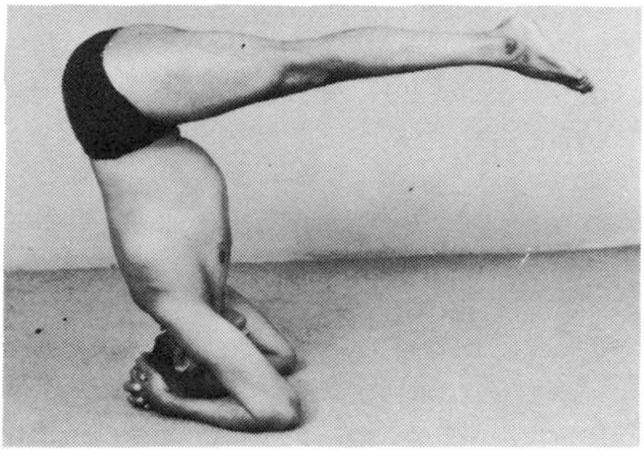

94

39. *Ūrdhvā Daṇḍāsana* Eight* (Plate 94)
(Ūrdhvā=up, daṇḍ=a staff)
Stay in this position for 10 seconds with normal breathing.

6. Exhale, move the legs up as in Plate 95, and then pull them up to the vertical position. (Side view: Plate 96.) Stay in this pose from 1 to 5 minutes while breathing evenly.

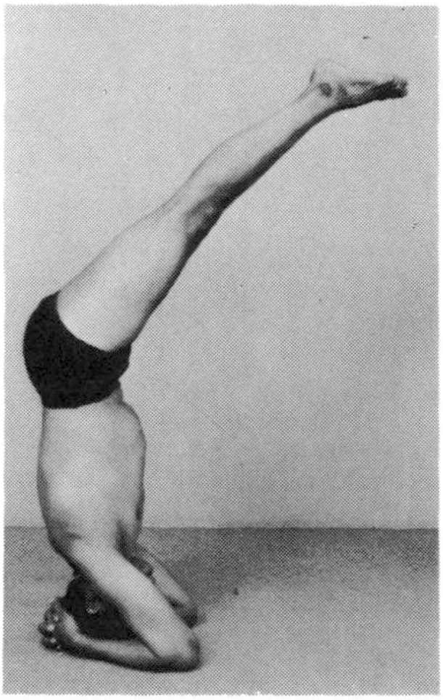
95

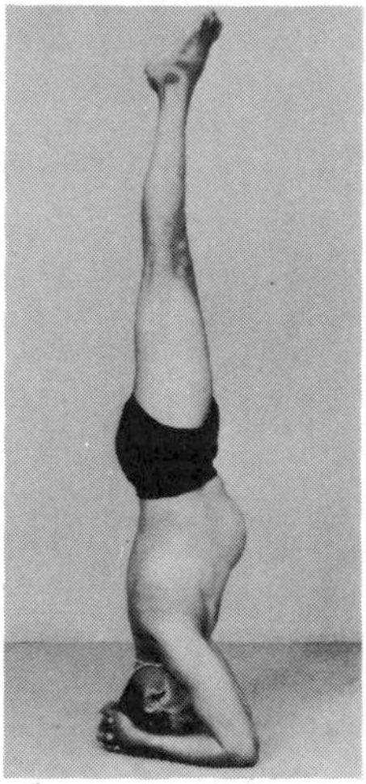
96

7. Come down gradually, observing the above technique in a reverse order. (Plates 95, 94, 93 and 92) Rest the feet on the floor, bend the knees (Plate 84) and raise the head from the floor or blanket. (Plate 83)

8. While coming down, it is advisable to stay in Ūrdhvā Daṇḍāsana according to capacity up to one minute while breathing normally. In this position, the neck and trunk will not be perpendicular to the floor but will sway slightly backwards. The neck, shoulders and spine will be put to a very great strain and in the initial stages one cannot stay with the legs parallel to the floor for more than a few seconds. The

stay will become longer as the neck, shoulders, abdomen and spine become stronger.

Hints on Śīrṣāsana

1. In Śīrṣāsana the balance alone is not important. One has to watch from moment to moment and find out the subtle adjustments. When we stand on our feet, we need no extra effort, strength or attention, for the position is natural. Yet the correct method of standing affects our bearing and carriage. It is, therefore, necessary to master the correct method as pointed out in the note on Tāḍāsana. In Śīrṣāsana also, the correct position should be mastered, as a faulty posture in this āsana will lead to pains in the head, neck and back.

2. The whole weight of the body should be borne on the head alone and not on the forearms and hands. The forearms and hands are to be used only for support to check any loss of balance. In a good pose you feel a circle, about the size of an Indian rupee, of the head in contact with the blanket on the floor.

3. The back of the head, the trunk, the back of the thighs and the heels should be in a line perpendicular to the floor and not inclined to one side. The throat, chin and breast-bone should be in one line, otherwise the head will tilt to one side or move forward. As regards the interlocked hands behind the head, the palms should not be stuck into the head. The upper and the lower sides of the palms should be in a line, otherwise the crown of the head will not rest on the floor correctly.

4. The elbows and the shoulders should be in a line and the elbows should not be widened. The shoulders should be kept as high above the floor as possible by moving them up and stretching them sideways. In order to learn the correct shoulder stretch, release the interlocked fingers and remove the hands from behind the head and widen the wrists from the forearms, keeping the elbows stationary. Place the wrists

on the floor with the palms facing up, touch the shoulders with the fingers, keeping the wrists on the floor and maintain the balance. (Plate 97) This will not only improve the balance but also prepare you for the other Śīrṣāsana poses described later.

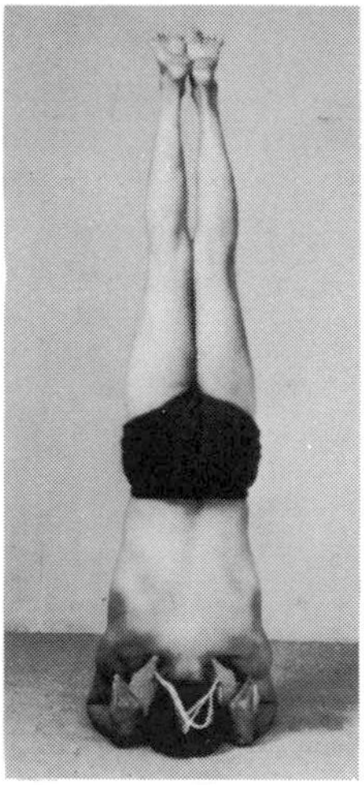

97

5. As to the position of the trunk, the dorsal region should be pushed forward as well as up. The lumbar (waist) and pelvic regions should not be pushed forward, while the trunk from the shoulders to the pelvis should be kept perpendicular. If the pelvic area juts forward, it means that you are bearing the weight of the body not on the head alone but also on the elbows for you have not stretched the dorsal region (the chest) correctly. When viewed from the side, the body from the neck to the heels should appear straight.

6. As far as possible try and join the thighs, knees, ankles and toes. Stretch the legs fully, especially the back of the knees and thighs. If the legs swing back tighten the knees and the lower median portion of the abdomen above the pubes. This will keep the legs perpendicular. Keep the toes pointing up. If the legs swing forward, stretch the dorsal region and

push the pelvic area slightly back until it is in line with the shoulders. The body will then feel light and the pose will be exhilarating.

7. While going up or holding the head stand the eyes should never become bloodshot. If they do, the pose is faulty.[1]

8. The time limit for Śīrṣāsana depends upon individual capacity and the time at one's disposal. One can hold it comfortably from 10 to 15 minutes. A beginner can do it for 2 minutes and go up to 5 minutes. It is always difficult for a beginner to balance for one minute, but once he succeeds he can be sure that from then on he will be able to master Śīrṣāsana soon.

9. While going up or coming down, move both legs together, inch by inch. All the movements should be done with exhalation. Inhale while waiting in a position. The effect of going down and coming up straight without bending the legs at the knees is that harmonious slow movement is gained and the flow of blood to the head is controlled. The face does not flush from jerky and fast movements, as the flow of blood to the waist and the legs is also controlled. Then there is no danger of losing balance from giddiness or numbness of the feet when one stands up immediately after the head balance. In course of time the whole movement of going up, staying and coming down should become as effortless as possible. In a perfect Śīrṣāsana your body feels completely stretched and at the same time you experience a feeling of complete relaxation.

10. It is always safe to perfect Sarvāngāsana (Plate 102) first before attempting Śīrṣāsana. If the standing poses described

[1] I have taught this pose to a lady of 65 who was suffering from glaucoma. Now she finds the eyes are completely rested and the pain in them is much lessened. Medical examination revealed that the tension in the eyeballs had decreased. I am mentioning this to prove the value of the correct head stand.

earlier (Plates 1 to 18) and the various movements of Sarvangāsana and Halāsana (Plates 108 to 125) are mastered first, Śīrṣāsana will come without much effort. If these elementary āsanas have not been mastered, the period taken to learn Śīrṣāsana will be longer.

11. After one has learnt to balance in Śīrṣāsana, however, it is preferable to perform Śīrṣāsana first before practising any other āsana. This is because one cannot balance or hold the head stand if the body is exhausted by doing other poses or if the breathing becomes fast and shaky. Once the body is tired or the breathing is not free and easy, the body will shake and it will be difficult to maintain the balance. It is always better to do Śīrṣāsana first when one is fresh.

12. Śīrṣāsana should always be followed by Sarvāngāsana and its cycle. It has been observed that people who devote themselves to Śīrṣāsana alone without doing the Sarvāngāsana poses are apt to lose their temper over trifling things and become irritated quickly. The practice of Sarvāngāsana coupled with Śīrṣāsana checks this trait. If Sarvāngāsana is the Mother, then Śīrṣāsana may be regarded as the Father of all āsanas. And just as both parents are necessary for peace and harmony in a home, so the practice of both these āsanas is essential to keep the body healthy and the mind tranquil and peaceful.

Effects of Śīrṣāsana

The ancient books have called Śīrṣāsana the king of all āsanas and the reasons are not hard to find. When we are born, normally the head comes out first and then the limbs. The skull encases the brain, which controls the nervous system and the organs of sense. The brain is the seat of intelligence, knowledge, discrimination, wisdom and power. It is the seat of Brahman, the soul. A country cannot prosper without a proper king or constitutional head to guide it; so also the human body cannot prosper without a healthy brain.

The *Bhagavad-Gītā* says: 'Harmony (sattva), mobility (rajas), inertia (tamas), such are the qualities, matter-born;

they bind fast, O great armed one (Arjuna), the indestructible dweller in the body.' (Fourteenth Discourse, verse 5) All these qualities stem from the brain, and sometimes one quality prevails and sometimes the others. The head is the centre of sattvic qualities which control discrimination; the trunk of Rājasic qualities which control passion, emotion and actions; and the region below the diaphragm of tāmasic qualities which control sensual pleasures like the enjoyment of food and drink, and the thrills and pleasures of sex.

Regular practice of Śīrṣāsana makes healthy pure blood flow through the brain cells. This rejuvenates them so that thinking power increases and thoughts become clearer. The āsana is a tonic for people whose brains tire quickly. It ensures a proper blood supply to the pituitary and pineal glands in the brain. Our growth, health and vitality depend on the proper functioning of these two glands.

People suffering from loss of sleep, memory and vitality have recovered by the regular and correct practice of this āsana and have become fountains of energy. The lungs gain the power to resist any climate and stand up to any work, which relieves one from colds, coughs, tonsilitis, halitosis (foul breath) and palpitations. It keeps the body warm. Coupled with Sarvāngāsana movements (Plates 108 to 125), it is a boon to people suffering from constipation. Regular practice of Śīrṣāsana will show marked improvement in the haemoglobin content of the blood.

It is not advisable to start with Śīrṣāsana and Sarvāngāsana when one suffers from high or low blood pressure.

Regular and precise practice of Śīrṣāsana develops the body, disciplines the mind and widens the horizons of the spirit. One becomes balanced and self-reliant in pain and pleasure, loss and gain, shame and fame and defeat and victory.

40. *Sālamba Sarvāngāsana I* Two* (Plates 102, 103 and 108)

Ālamba means a prop, a support and sa together with or accompanied by. Sālamba, therefore, means supported or propped up. Sarvānga (Sarva=all, whole, entire, complete; anga=limb or body) means the entire body or all the limbs.

In this pose the whole body benefits from the exercise, hence the name.

Technique for beginners

1. Lie flat on the back on the carpet keeping the legs stretched out, tightened at the knees. Place the hands by the side of the legs, palms down. (Plate 98) Take a few deep breaths.

2. Exhale, bend the knees and move the legs towards the stomach till the thighs press it. (Plate 99) Take two breaths.

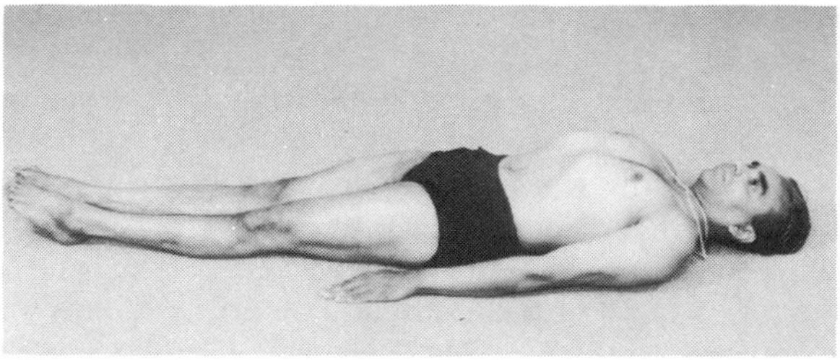

98

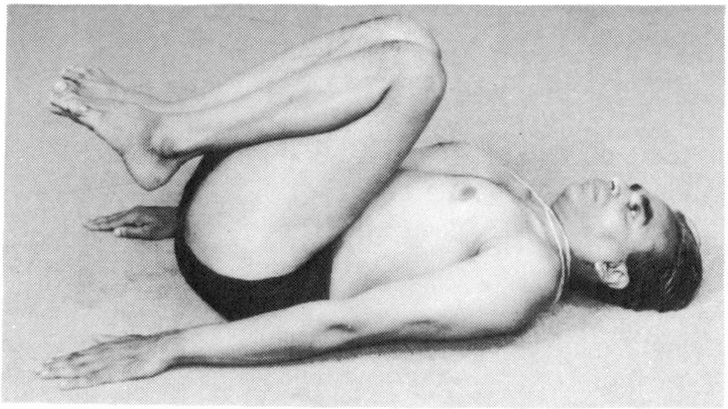

99

3. Raise the hips from the floor with an exhalation and rest the hands on them by bending the arms at the elbows. (Plate 100) Take two breaths.

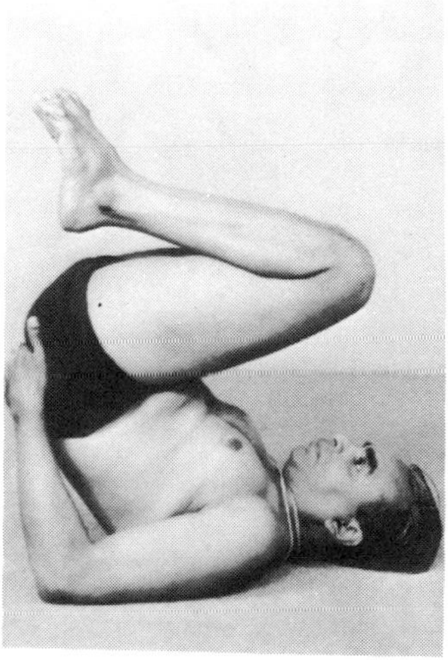

100

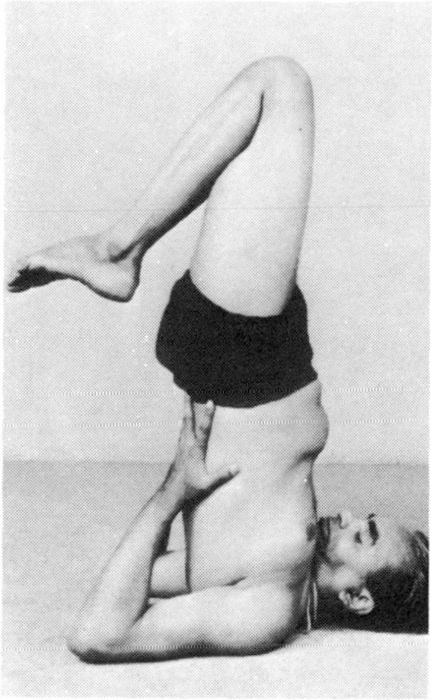

101

4. Exhale, raise the trunk up perpendicularly supported by the hands until the chest touches the chin. (Plate 101)

5. Only the back of the head and the neck, the shoulders and the backs of the arms up to the elbows should rest on the floor. Place the hands in the middle of the spine as in Plate 101. Take two breaths.

6. Exhale and stretch the legs straight with the toes pointing up. (Front view: Plate 102. Back view: Plate 103)

7. Stay in this position for 5 minutes with even breathing.

8. Exhale, gradually slide down, release the hands, lie flat and relax.

9. If you cannot do the āsana without support use a stool and follow the technique. See Plate 104.

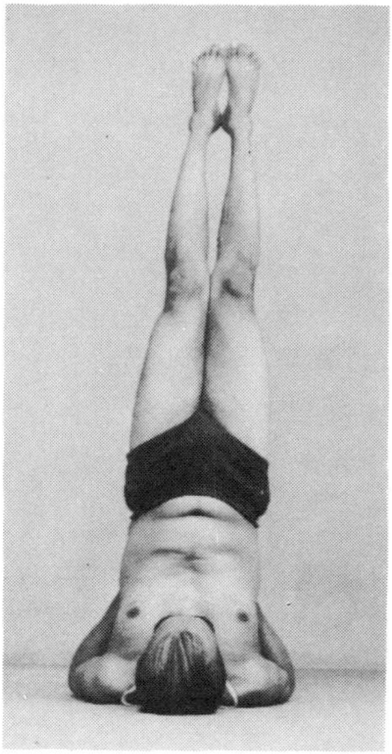

102

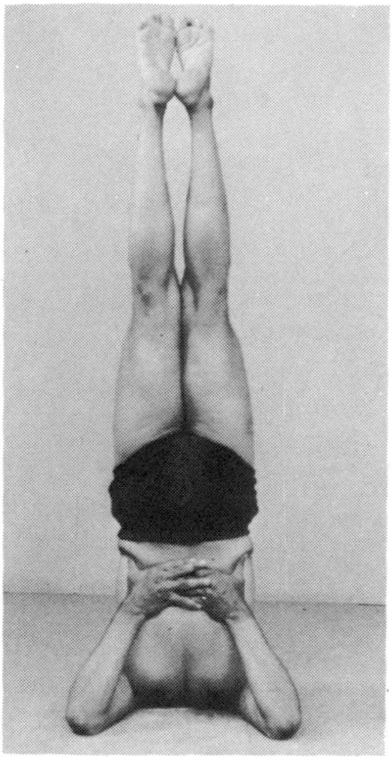

103

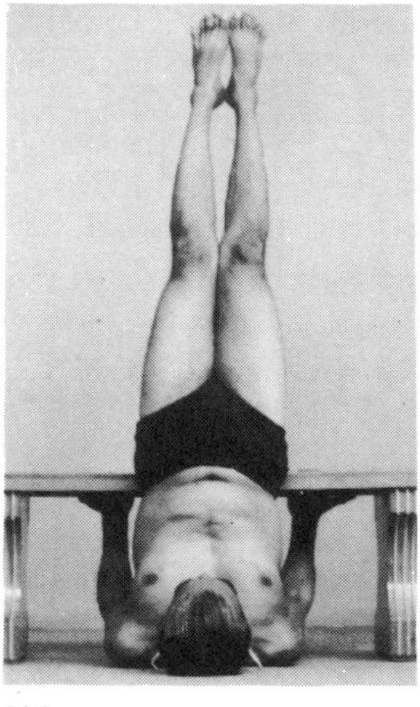

104

Technique for advanced pupils

1. Lie flat on the back on the carpet.

2. Keep the legs stretched out, tightened at the knees. Place the hands by the side of the legs, palms down. (Plate 98)

3. Take a few deep breaths. Exhale slowly and at the same time raise both legs together and bring them at a right angle to the body. (Plate 105) Remain in this position and inhale, keeping the legs steady.

4. Exhale, again raise the legs further up by lifting the hips and back from the floor, pressing the palms gently against the floor as in Plate 106.

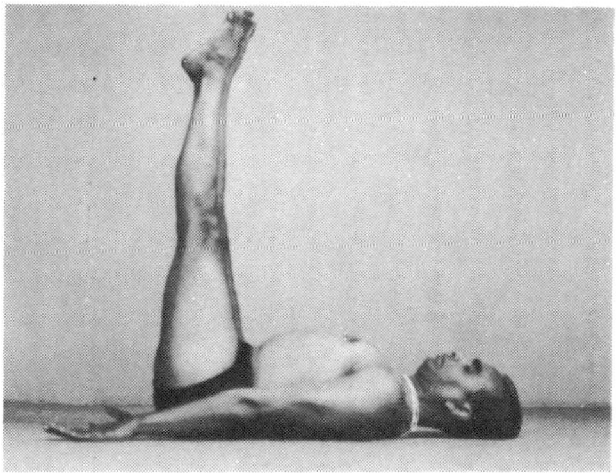

105

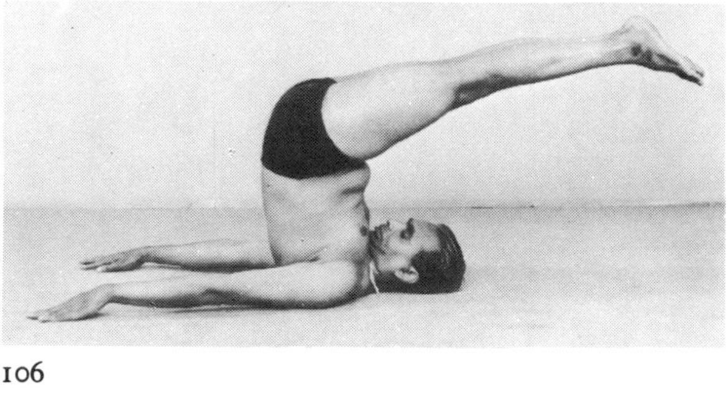

106

5. When the whole trunk is raised off the ground, bend the elbows and place the palms on the back of the ribs, resting the shoulders well on the floor.

6. Utilise the palm pressure and raise the trunk and legs up vertically as in Plate 107 so that the breast-bone presses the chin to form a firm chinlock. The contraction of the throat and pressing the chin against the breast-bone to form a firm chinlock is known as Jālandhara Bandha. Remember to bring the chest forward to touch the chin and not to bring the chin towards the chest. If the latter is done, the spine is not stretched completely and the full effect of this āsana will not be felt.

7. Only the back of the head and neck, the shoulders and the upper portion of the arms up to the elbows should rest well on the floor. The remainder of the body should be in one straight line, perpendicular to the floor. This is the final position. (Side view: Plate 108)

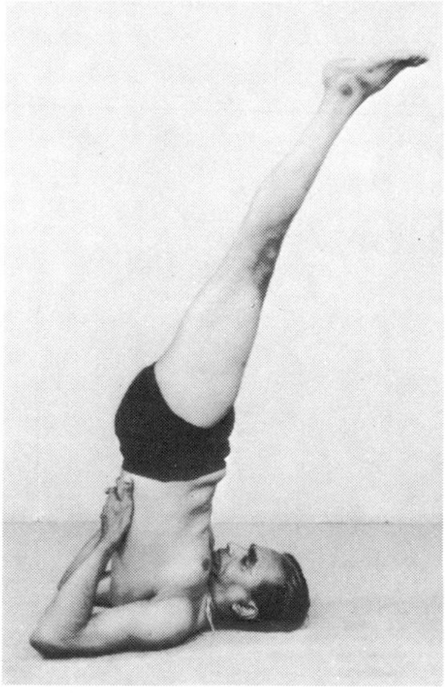

107

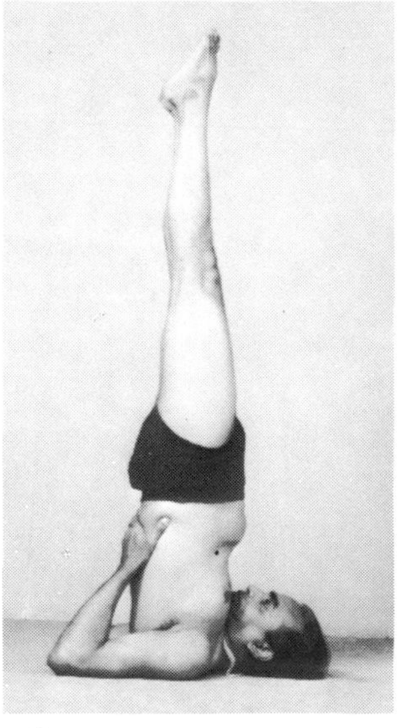

108

8. In the beginning, there is a tendency for the legs to swing out of the perpendicular. To correct this, tighten the back thigh muscles and stretch up vertically.

9. The elbows should not be placed wider than the shoulders. Try and stretch the shoulders away from the neck and also to bring the elbows close to each other. If the elbows are widened, the trunk cannot be pulled up properly and the pose will look imperfect. Also see that the neck is straight with the centre of the chin resting on the sternum. In the beginning, the neck moves sideways and if this is not corrected, it will cause pain and injure the neck.

10. Remain in this pose for not less than 5 minutes. Gradually increase the time to 15 minutes; this will have no ill effects.

11. Release the hands, slide down to the floor, lie flat and relax.

As the weight of the whole body is borne on the neck and shoulders and as the hands are used to support the weight this āsana is called Sālamba Sarvāngāsana. In Sarvāngāsana there are various movements which can be done in addition to the basic pose described above.

Effects

The importance of Sarvāngāsana cannot be overemphasised. It is one of the greatest boons conferred on humanity by our ancient sages. Sarvāngāsana is the Mother of āsanas. As a mother strives for harmony and happiness in the home, so this āsana strives for the harmony and happiness of the human system. It is a panacea for most common ailments. There are several endocrine organs or ductless glands in the human system which bathe in blood, absorb the nutriments from the blood and secrete hormones for the proper functioning of a balanced and well developed body and brain. If the glands fail to function properly, the hormones are not produced as they should be and the body starts to deteriorate. Amazingly enough many of the āsanas have a direct effect on the glands and help them to function properly. Sarvāngāsana does this for the thyroid and parathyroid glands which are situated in the neck region, since due to the firm chinlock their blood supply is increased. Further, since the body is inverted the venous blood flows to the heart without any strain by force of gravity. Healthy blood is allowed to circulate around the neck and chest. As a result, persons suffering from breathlessness, palpitation, asthma, bronchitis and throat ailments get relief. As the head remains firm in this inverted position, and the supply of the blood to it is regulated by the firm chinlock, the nerves are soothed and headaches – even chronic ones - disappear. Continued practice of this āsana eradicates common colds and other nasal disturbances. Due to the soothing effect of the pose on the nerves, those suffering from hypertension, irritation, shortness of temper, nervous breakdown and insomnia are relieved. The change in bodily gravity also affects the abdominal organs so that the bowels move freely and constipation vanishes. As a result the system is freed from toxins and one feels full of energy. The āsana is recommended for urinary disorders and uterine displacement, menstrual trouble, piles and hernia. It also helps to relieve epilepsy, low vitality and anaemia. It is no over-statement to say that if a person regularly practises Sarvāngāsana he will feel new vigour and strength, and will be happy and confident. New life will flow into him, his mind will be at peace and he will feel the joy of life. After a long illness, the practice of this āsana regularly twice a day brings back lost vitality. The Sarvāngāsana cycle activates the abdominal organs and relieves people suffering from stomach and intestinal ulcers, severe pains in the abdomen and colitis.

People suffering from high blood pressure should not attempt Sālamba Sarvāngāsana unless they do Halāsana (Plate 113) first and can stay in it for not less than 3 minutes.

Do not perform Sarvāngāsana during menstruation.

Halāsana is described on the following pages.

The Sarvāngāsana Cycle

These various movements can be practised at one stretch

after staying in Sarvāngāsana (Plate 102) from 5 to 10 minutes or more according to capacity; do them for 20 to 30 seconds at a time each side except Halāsana, which should last from 3 to 5 minutes at a stretch.

41. *Halāsana* Four* (Plate 113)

Hala means a plough, the shape of which this posture resembles, hence the name. It is a part of Sarvāngāsana I and a continuation thereof.

Technique

1. Do Sālamba Sarvāngāsana (Plate 103) with a firm chinlock.

2. Release the chinlock, lower the trunk slightly, moving the arms and legs over the head and resting the tóes on the floor. (Plate 109)

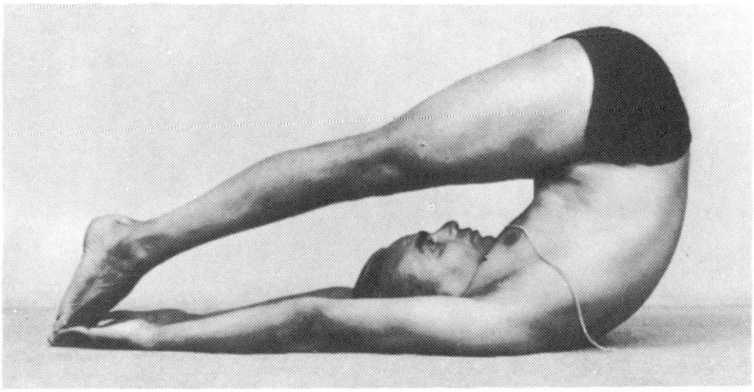

109

3. Tighten the knees by pulling up the hamstring muscles at the back of the thighs and raise the trunk. (Plate 110)

4. Stretch the arms on the floor in the direction opposite to that of the legs. (Plate 111)

5. Interlock the fingers (Plate 112) and turn the wrists so that the thumbs rest on the floor. (Plate 113) Stretch the palms

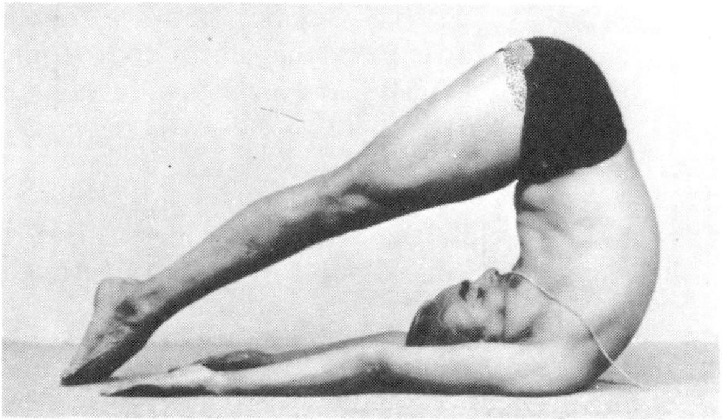

110

along with the fingers, tighten the arms at the elbows and pull them from the shoulders.

6. The legs and the hands are stretched in opposite directions and this stretches the spine completely.

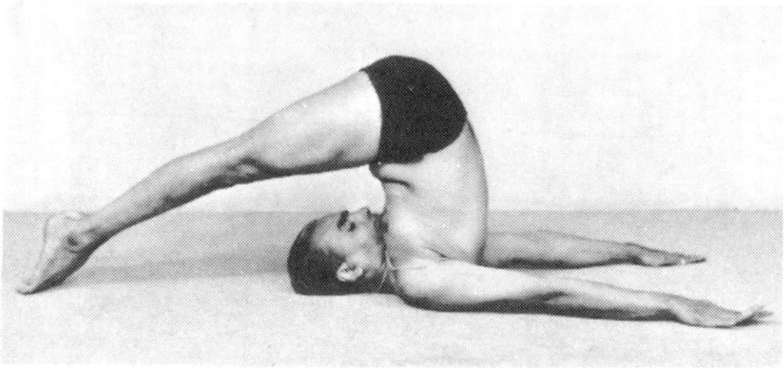

111

7. While interlocking the fingers, it is advisable to change the interlock. Suppose that the right thumb touches the floor first, maintain the position for a minute. Then release the grip and bring the left thumb first on the floor, follow the interlock, finger by finger, and stretch out the arms for the same length of time. This will lead to harmonious development and elasticity of both the shoulders, elbows and wrists.

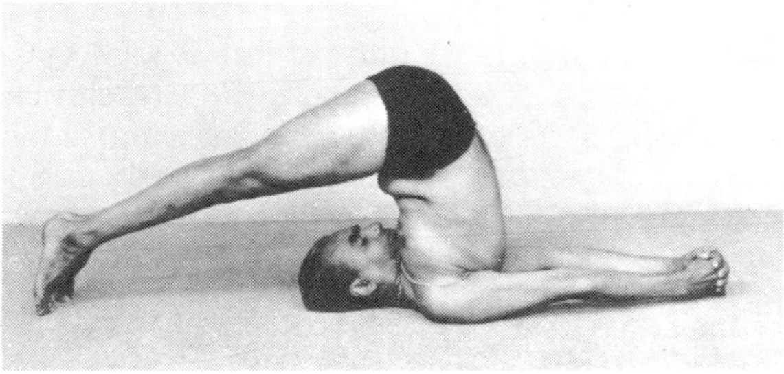

112

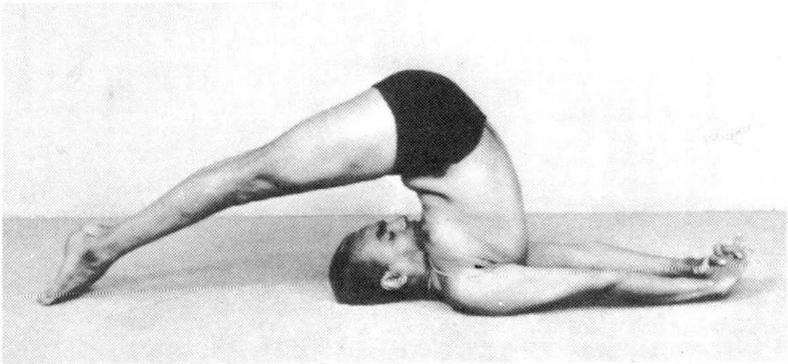

113

8. In the beginning interlocking will be difficult. By gradual practice of the above mentioned positions, you will interlock the fingers easily.

9. In the beginning it is also difficult to keep the toes firmly on the floor behind the head. If you lengthen the timing and stretch of Sarvāngāsana (Plate 102) before going into Halāsana, the toes will remain longer on the floor.

10. Remain in the attainable pose from one to five minutes with normal breathing.

11. Release the hands. Raise the legs up to Sarvāngāsana and gradually slide down to the floor. Lie flat on the back and relax.

Effects

The effect of Halāsana is the same as that of Sarvāngāsana. (Plate 102) In addition, the abdominal organs are rejuvenated due to contraction. The spine receives an extra supply of blood due to the forward bend and this helps to relieve backache. Cramps in the hands are cured by interlocking and stretching the palms and fingers. People suffering from stiff shoulders and elbows, lumbago and arthritis of the back find relief in this āsana. Griping pain in the stomach due to wind is also relieved and lightness is felt immediately.

The pose is good for people with a tendency for high blood pressure. If they perform Halāsana first and then Sarvāngāsana, they will not feel the rush of blood or the sensation of fullness in the head.

Halāsana is a preparatory pose to Paschimottānāsana. (Plate 81) If one improves in Halāsana, the resulting mobility of the back will enable one to perform Paschimottānāsana well.

Note: For persons suffering from high blood pressure the following technique is recommended for doing Halāsana before they attempt Sālamba Sarvāngāsana.

1. Lie flat on the back on the floor.

2. Exhale, slowly raise the legs to a perpendicular position and stay there breathing normally for about 10 seconds.

3. Exhale, bring the legs over and beyond the head and touch the toes on the floor. Keep the toes on the floor and the legs stiff at the knees.

4. If you have difficulty in keeping the toes on the floor, then place a chair or a stool behind the head and rest the toes on it.

5. If the breathing becomes heavy or fast do not rest the toes on the floor, but on a stool or chair. Then fullness or pressure is not felt in the head.

6. Extend the arms over the head, keep them on the floor and stay in this position with normal breathing for 3 minutes.

7. Throughout the āsana, gaze at the tip of the nose with the eyes shut.

42. *Karṇapīdāsana* One* (Plate 114b)
Karṇa means the ear. Pīda means pain, discomfort or pressure. This is a variant of Halāsana and can be done along with it.

Technique
1. Do Halāsana (Plate 113) and after completing the time limit for that pose, flex the knees and rest the right knee by the side of the right ear and the left knee by the side of the left.

2. Both knees should rest on the floor, pressing the ears.

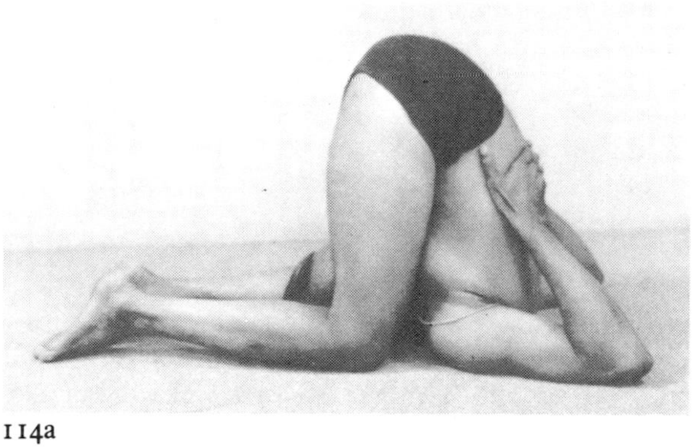

114a

3. Keep the toes stretched out and join the heels and toes. Rest the hands either on the back of the ribs (Plate 114a), or interlock the fingers and stretch out the arms (Plate 114b).

4. Remain in this position for half a minute or a minute with normal breathing.

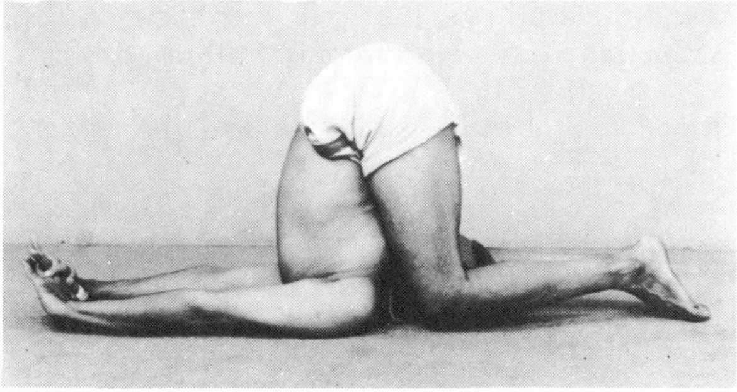

114b

Effects
This āsana rests the trunk, heart and legs. The spine is stretched more while bending the knees, and this helps the circulation of blood round the waistline.

43. *Supta Koṇāsana* Two* (Plate 115)
Supta means lying down and koṇa an angle. It is a variation of Halāsana in which the legs are spread apart.

Technique
1. From Karṇapīdāsana (Plates 114a, 114b), stretch the legs straight and spread the legs as far apart as you can.

2. Pull the trunk up and tighten the knees.

3. Hold the right toe with the right hand and the left toe with the left one. Keep the heels up. After gripping the toes, move the dorsal region of the spine still further up and extend the hamstring muscles. (Plate 115)

4. Stay in the pose from 20 to 30 seconds with normal breathing.

Effects
This pose tones the legs and helps to contract the abdominal organs.

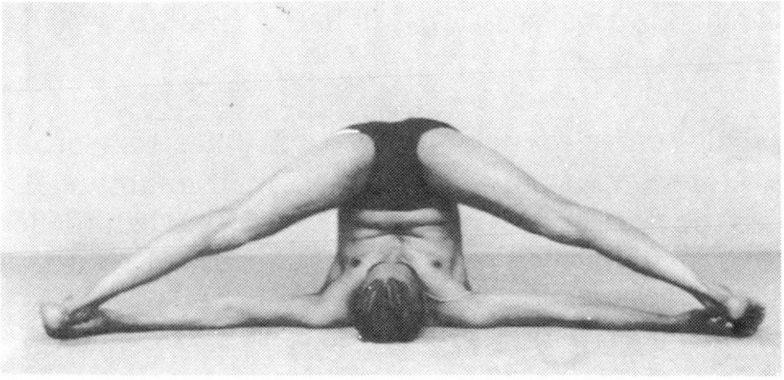

115

44. *Pārśva Halāsana* Four* (Plate 116)
In Halāsana (Plate 114) both the legs rest behind the head. In this pose they rest sideways on one side of and in line with the head. This is the lateral plough pose.

Technique

1. Do Supta Koṇāsana (Plate 115) and come back to Halāsana.

2. Place the palms on the back of the ribs.

3. Move both the legs as far as you can to the left.

4. Tighten both knees, raise the trunk up with the help of the palms and stretch the legs. (Plate 116)

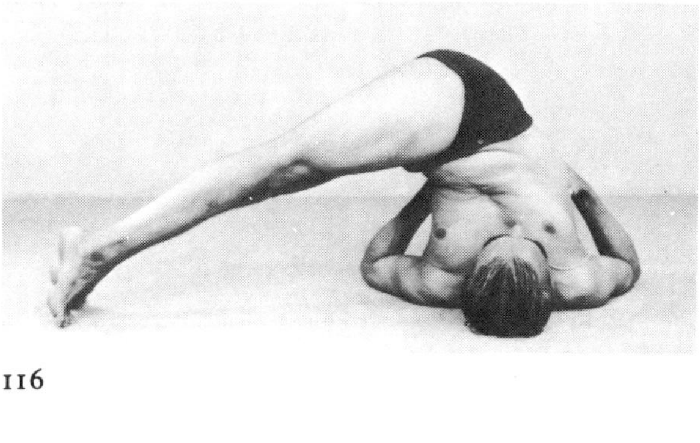

116

5. Remain in this position for half a minute with normal breathing.

6. Exhale, move the legs to the right until they are in line with the head and hold the pose for half a minute. Do not disturb the position of the chest and trunk when the legs are moved. The chest and trunk should remain as in Sarvāngāsana or Halāsana.

Effects

In this āsana, the spine moves laterally and becomes more elastic. The colon, which is inverted during the movements, is exercised properly and elimination will be complete. People suffering from acute or chronic constipation which is the mother of several diseases derive great benefit from this āsana. If rubbish is dumped outside our house we feel sick. How much more so when waste matter which creates toxins is allowed to accumulate in our own system? If this waste matter is not eliminated, diseases will enter the body like thieves and rob us of health. If the bowels do not move freely, the mind becomes dull and one feels heavy and irritable. This āsana helps us keep the bowels free and thereby win the prize of health.

45. *Eka Pāda Sarvāngāsana* Five* (Plate 117)

Eka means one, single. Pāda means the foot. In this variation of Sarvāngāsana, one leg is on the floor in Halāsana, while the other is in a vertical position along with the trunk.

Technique

1. Do Sālamba Sarvāngāsana I. (Plate 102)

2. Keep the left leg up in Sarvāngāsana. Exhale and move the right leg down to the floor to Halāsana. (Plate 117) It should remain stiff and straight and not bend at the knee. If it is not possible to touch the floor, lower the leg as far as possible.

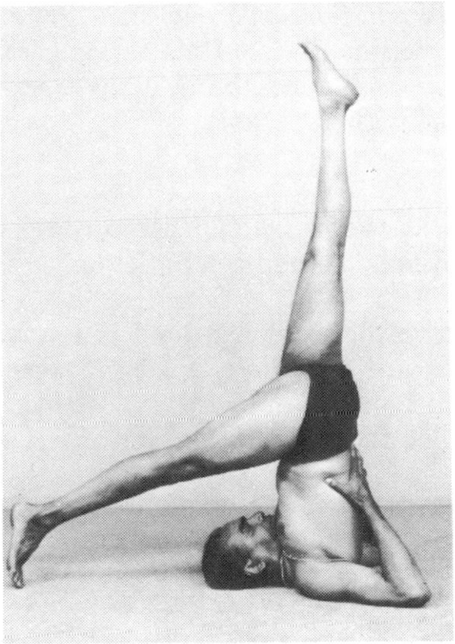

117

3. While resting the right leg on the floor, the left knee should be kept taut and not allowed to tilt sideways. The left leg should be kept straight, facing the head.

4. Stay in the pose for 20 seconds maintaining normal breathing.

5. Exhale, lift the right leg back to Sarvāngāsana, and then move the left leg down to the floor in Halāsana, keeping the right leg vertically up and stiff. Lifting the leg from the floor back to Sarvāngāsana exercises the abdominal organs more than if one brings both legs down to Halāsana.

6. Stay on this side for the same length of time.

Effects
This āsana tones the kidneys and the leg muscles.

46. *Pārśvaika Pāda Sarvāngāsana* Six* (Plate 118)
Pārśva means the side. In Eka Pāda Sarvāngāsana (Plate 117) the lower leg rests behind the head, whereas here it rests sideways in line with the trunk.

Technique

1. Perform Eka Pāda Sarvāngāsana on both sides as described above and come back to Sarvāngāsana.

2. Exhale, move the right leg down sideways to the floor until it is in line with the trunk. (Plate 118) Keep the right leg straight and stiff and do not bend it at the knee. If it is not possible to touch the floor, lower the leg as far as possible.

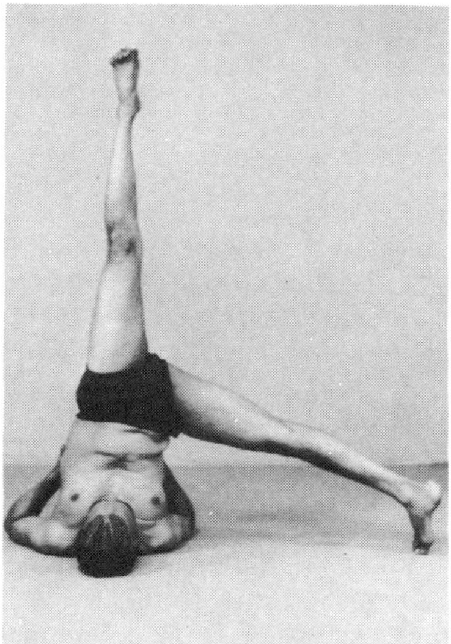

118

3. The left leg which is vertically up should be kept straight and not allowed to tilt to the right. The ribs should be lifted with the palms to expand the chest fully.

4. Remain in the pose for 20 seconds with normal breathing, exhale, and go back to Sarvāngāsana. Repeat with the other leg for the same length of time and return to Sarvāngāsana.

Effects

This pose relieves constipation and also tones the kidneys.

47. *Setu Bandha Sarvāngāsana* – also called *Uttāna Mayūrāsana* Ten* (Plate 121)

Setu means a bridge and Setu Bandha means the formation or construction of a bridge. In this position, the body is arched and supported on the shoulders, soles and heels. The arch is supported by the hands at the waist.

Ut means intense and tān means to stretch. This āsana resembles a stretched peacock (Mayūra), hence the name.

Technique

1. Do Sālamba Sarvāngāsana. (Plate 102)

2. Rest the palms well on the back, raise the spine up, bend the knees (Plate 119) and throw the legs back over the wrists to the floor. (Plate 120) Stretch out the legs and keep them together. (Plate 121)

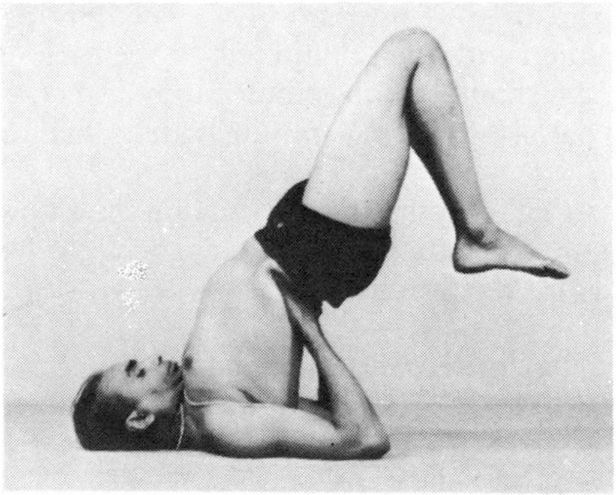

119

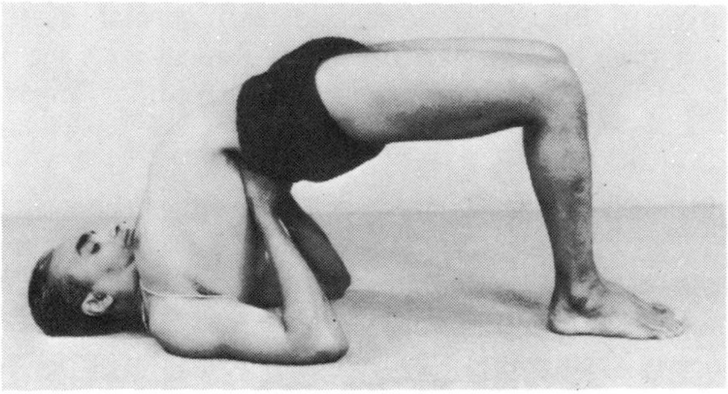

120

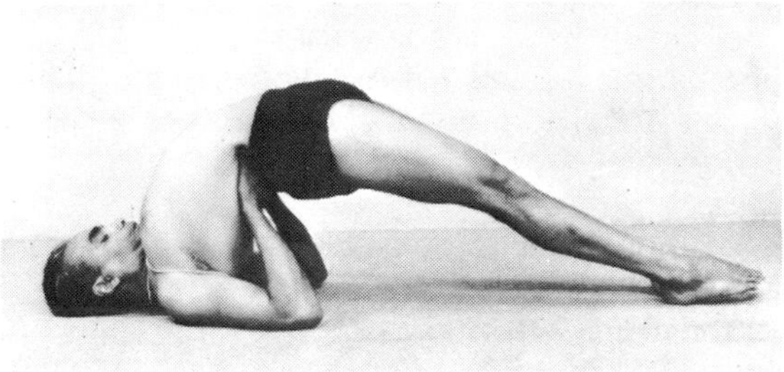

121

3. The whole body forms a bridge, the weight of which is borne by the elbows and the wrists. The only parts of the body in contact with the ground will be the back of the head and neck, the shoulders, the elbows and the feet. Stay in the pose from half a minute to a minute with normal breathing.

4. It is possible to lessen the pressure on the elbows and the wrists by stretching the spine towards the neck, keeping the heels firmly on the ground.

Effects of Setu Bandha Sarvāngāsana

This āsana gives the spine a backward movement and removes the strain on the neck caused by the other various movements of Sarvāngāsana.

A healthy and flexible spine indicates a healthy nervous

system. If the nerves are healthy a man is sound in mind and body.

48. *Ūrdhva Padmāsana in Sarvāngāsana* Four* (Plate 122)
Ūrdhva means above, high. Padma means a lotus. In this Sarvāngāsana variation, the legs, instead of being kept straight up, are bent at the knees and crossed so that the right foot rests on the left thigh and the left foot on the right thigh as in the lotus pose. (Plate 53)

Technique

1. From Sālamba Sarvāngāsana, bend the legs at the knees and cross them. First place the right foot over the left thigh, and then the left foot over the right thigh.

2. Stretch the crossed legs vertically up, move the knees closer to each other and the legs as far back as possible from the pelvic region. (Plate 122)

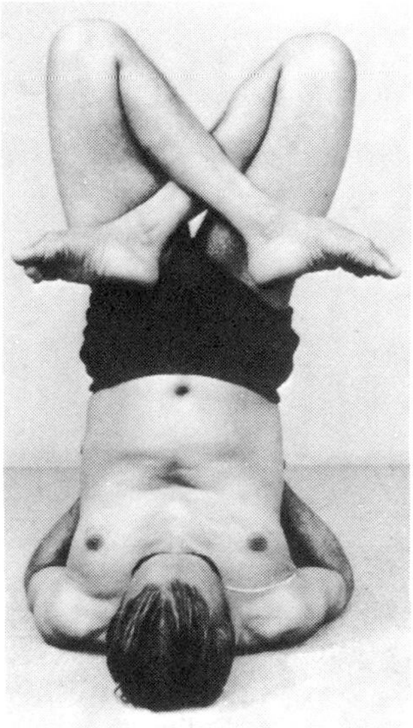

122

3. Stay in this pose from 20 to 30 seconds with deep and even breathing.

4. Uncross the legs, return to Sālamba Sarvāngāsana and repeat the pose by first placing the left foot over the right thigh and then the right foot over the left thigh. Stay for an equal length of time in all these positions as in the earlier ones.

49. *Pinḍāsana in Sarvāngāsana* Five* (Plate 123)
Pinḍa means embryo or foetus. In this variation of Sarvāngāsana which is a continuation of the earlier posture, the bent crossed legs are brought down until they rest on the head. The posture resembles that of an embryo in the womb, hence the name.

Technique
1. From Ūrdhva Padmāsana in Sarvāngāsana (Plate 122), exhale, bend and lower the crossed legs from the hips towards the head.

2. Rest the legs over the head. (Plate 123)

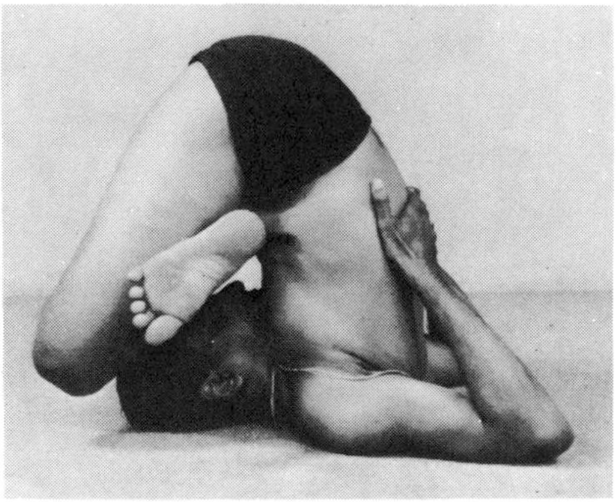

123

3. Remain in this position from 20 to 30 seconds with normal breathing and go back to Ūrdhva Padmāsana in Sarvāngāsana.

50. *Pārśva Piṇḍāsana in Sarvāngāsana* Eight* (Plates 124 and 125) Pārśva means the side or flank. In this Piṇḍāsana variation of the earlier pose, both the bent knees are moved sideways and placed on the floor on the same side of the trunk. This is the lateral embryo pose in Sarvāngāsana.

Technique

1. After staying in Pindāsana (Plate 123) turn the hips sideways to the right, exhale and lower both knees to the floor. The left knee should be by the side of the right ear. (Plate 124)

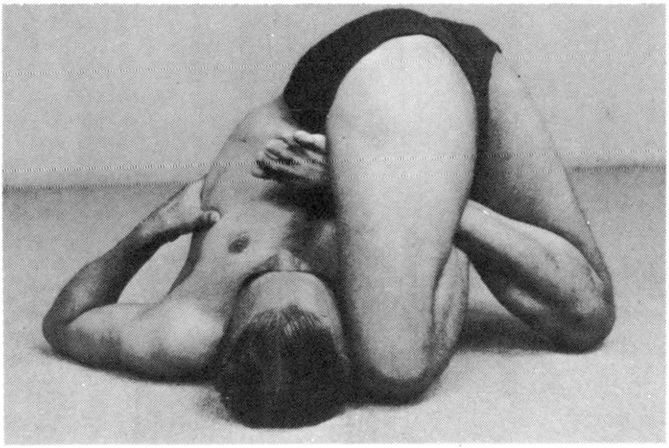

124

2. The left shoulder will be raised off the floor in the beginning. Push the shoulder against the floor and press the left hand firmly against the back. If this is not done, you will lose balance and roll over to one side.

3. Due to the lateral twist, breathing will be fast and difficult as the diaphragm is pressed in this position.

4. The knee near the ear will not rest on the floor to start with, but only after long practice.

5. Stay in this position for 20 to 30 seconds, with normal breathing.

6. Exhale, come up from the right side and move the crossed legs over to the left, so that the left foot will be near the left ear. (Plate 125) Stay here also for the same length of time.

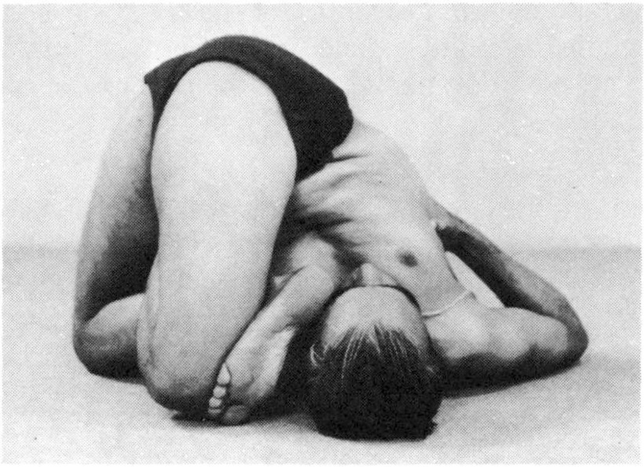

125

7. Go back to Ūrdhva Padmāsana. (Plate 122) Release the lotus pose by uncrossing the legs and return to Sālamba Sarvāngāsana.

8. Now change the position of the crossed legs. Cross the legs again by putting the left foot over the right thigh first and then the right foot over the left thigh instead of the other way as done earlier.

9. Repeat the movements again on both the sides as described earlier.

Effects of Ūrdhva Padmāsana and Pārśva Piṇḍāsana movements in Sarvāngāsana

The change of crossing the legs brings equal pressure on both sides of the abdomen and colon and relieves constipation. For those suffering from chronic constipation a longer stay in Pārśva Piṇḍāsana is recommended, and one minute on each side will prove most efficacious. Griping pain in the stomach is relieved by these poses.

Persons with extremely flexible knees, can easily perform these positions. It is, however, difficult for many people to cross the legs in Padmāsana. For them a longer stay in Pārśva Halāsana (Plate 116) – (there also the spine and trunk get a lateral twist but the legs remain straight) – is recommended.

In all these positions breathing at first will be fast and laboured. Try to maintain normal breathing.

Note. The spine is given the forward, lateral and backward movements in these variations of Sarvāngāsana. In Halāsana, Eka Pāda Sarvāngāsana, Karṇa Pīdāsana and Piṇḍāsana the spine moves in the forward direction. In Pārśvaika Pāda Sarvānga, Pārśva Halāsana and Pārśva Piṇḍāsana the spine moves laterally. In Setu Bandha it is given a backward movement. These movements tone the spine on all sides and keep it healthy.

It is related that in the Krita Age (the first Age of the Universe) a host of Dānavās (giants and demons) became invincible in battle under the leadership of Vṛtra and scattered the Devas (or Gods) in all directions. Realising that they could not regain their power until Vṛtra was destroyed, the gods appeared before their Grandsire, Brahmā, the creator. Brahmā instructed them to consult Viṣṇu who asked them to obtain the bones of a sage called Dadhīcha, from which to make a demon-slaying weapon. The gods appeared before the sage and begged the boon according to Viṣṇu's advice. The sage renounced his body for the benefit of the gods. From the spine of Dadhīcha was fashioned Vajra, the thunderbolt, which Indra the king of the gods hurled and slew Vṛtra.

The story is symbolical. The Dānavās represent the

tāmasic qualities in men and diseases. The Devas represent health, harmony and peace. To destroy the tāmasic qualities and the diseases due to them and to enjoy health and happiness, we have to make our spines strong as a thunderbolt like the spine of Dadhīcha. Then we shall enjoy health, harmony and happiness in abundance.

51. *Jaṭara Parivartanāsana* Five* (Plates 127 and 128)Jaṭara means the stomach, the belly. Parivartana means turning or rolling about, turning round.

Technique

1. Lie flat on the back on the floor. (Plate 98)

2. Exhale, raise both legs together until they are perpendicular to the floor. They should remain poker stiff, so do not bend them at the knees. (Plate 105)

3. Stretch out both arms sideways in line with the shoulders, so that the body resembles a cross.

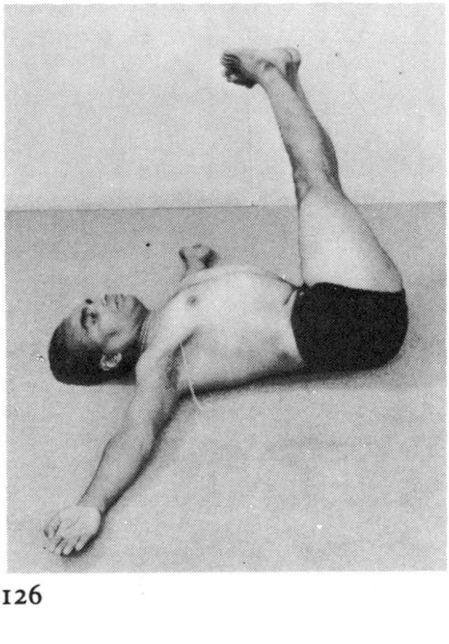

126

4. Remain in this position for a few breaths. Then exhale, and move both the legs sideways (Plate 126) down towards the floor to the left until the toes of the left foot almost touch the finger-tips of the outstretched left hand. (Plate 127) Try and keep the back well on the floor. In the initial stages, the right shoulder will be lifted off the floor. To prevent this ask a friend to press it down, or catch hold of a heavy piece of furniture with the right hand when the legs are turned sideways to the left.

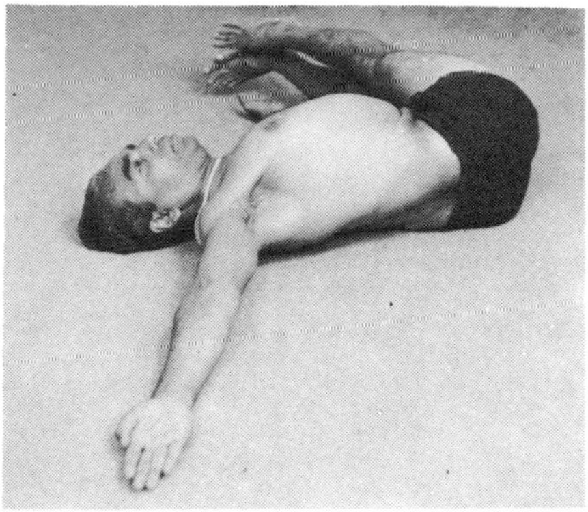

127

5. Both legs should go down together, the knees being kept tight throughout. As far as possible keep the lumbar portion of the back on the floor and turn the legs only from the hips. When the legs are near the outstretched left hand, move the abdomen to the right.

6. Stay in the pose for about 20 seconds, keeping the legs stiff throughout. Then move the still stiffened legs slowly back to the perpendicular with an exhalation.

7. Remain with the legs perpendicular for a few breaths and then repeat the movements by lowering the legs to the right and turning the abdomen to the left. (Plate 128) Stay here

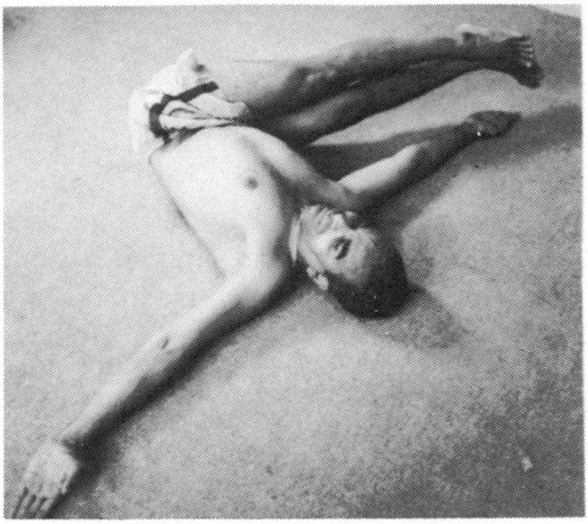

128

also for the same length of time and with an exhalation, come back to the perpendicular legs position and then gently lower the legs to the floor (Plate 98) and relax.

Effects
This āsana is good for reducing excess fat. It tones and eradicates sluggishness of the liver, spleen and pancreas. It also cures gastritis and strengthens the intestines. By its regular practice all the abdominal organs are kept in trim. It helps to relieve sprains and catches in the lower back and the hip region.

52. *Supta Pādānguṣṭhāsana* Thirteen* (Plate 130)
Supta means lying down. Pāda is the foot. Anguṣṭha means the big toe. Hence the name.

Technique
1. Lie flat on the back, stretch both legs and keep the knees tight. (Plate 98)

2. Inhale, raise the left leg from the floor until it is perpendicular. Keep the right leg stretched fully on the floor and rest the right hand on the right thigh.

3. Raise the left arm and catch the left big toe between the thumb and the fore and middle fingers. (Plate 129) Take 3 or 4 deep breaths.

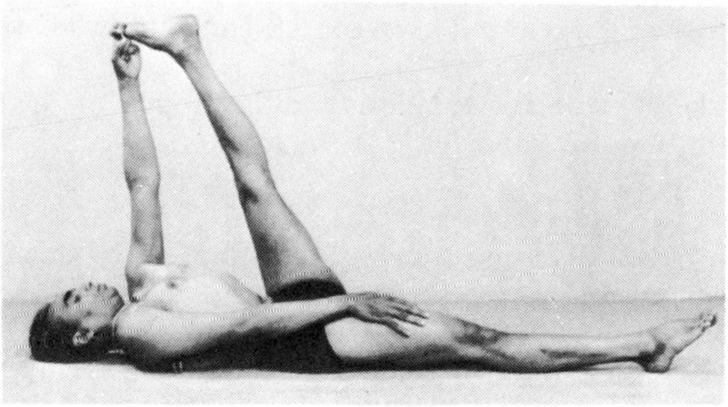

129

4. Exhale, raise the head and trunk from the floor, bend the left arm at the elbow and pull the left leg towards the head without bending it at the knee. Pull the leg down, lift the head and trunk up together and rest the chin on the left knee. (Plate 130) Stay in this position for about 20 seconds, keeping the right leg fully stretched straight along the floor while breathing normally.

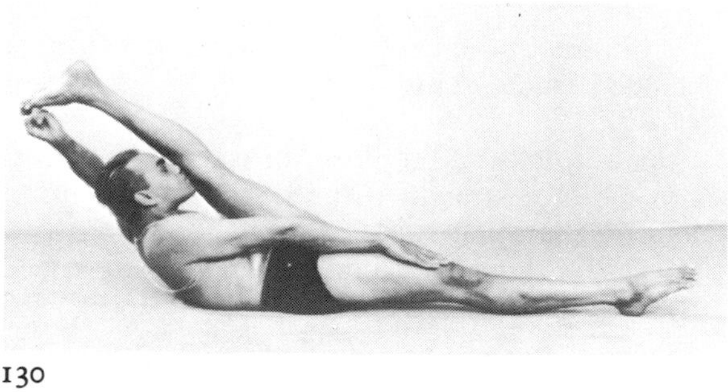

130

5. Inhale, move the head and trunk back to the floor and the left leg back to the perpendicular. (Plate 129) This completes the first movement.

6. Exhale, release the toe grip, rest the left leg on the floor beside the right one and keep the left hand on the left thigh.

7. Take a few deep inhalations and then repeat on the right, substituting the word 'left' for the word 'right'.

Effects
The legs will develop properly by the practice of this āsana. Persons suffering from sciatica and paralysis of the legs will derive great benefit from it. The blood is made to circulate in the legs and hips where the nerves are rejuvenated The pose removes stiffness in the hip joints and prevents hernia. It can be practised by both men and women.

53. *Bharadvājāsana* One* (Plates 131 and 132)
Bharadvāja was the father of Droṇa, the military preceptor of the Kauravas and Pāṇḍavas, who fought the great war described in the Mahābhārata. This āsana is dedicated to Bharadvāja.

Technique
1. Sit on the floor with the legs stretched straight in front. (Plate 35)

2. Flex the knees, move the legs back and bring both feet to the right side beside the hip.

3. Rest the buttocks on the floor, turn the trunk about 45 degrees to the left, straighten the right arm and place the right hand on the outer side of the left thigh near the left knee. Insert the right hand underneath the left knee, the palm touching the floor.

4. Exhale, turn the left arm from the shoulder behind the

back, bend the left elbow and with the left hand clasp the right upper arm above the right elbow.

5. Turn the neck to the right and gaze over the right shoulder. (Plates 131 and 132)

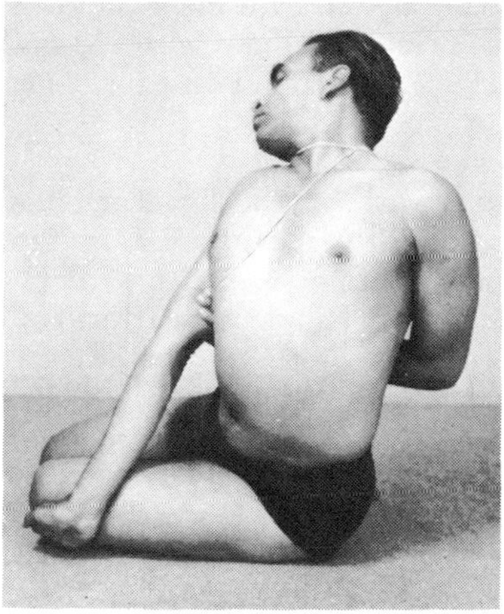

131

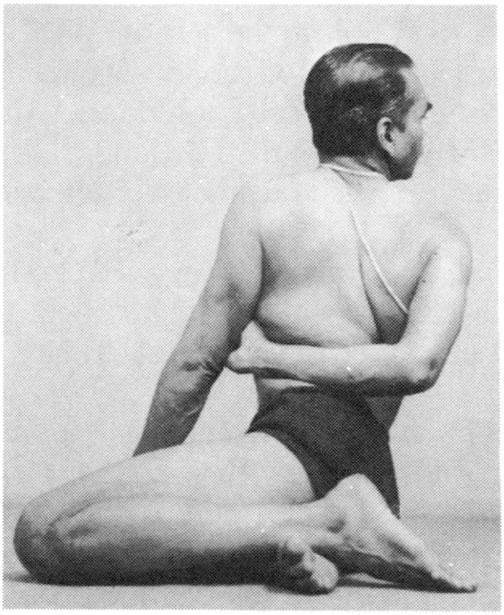

132

6. Hold the position for half a minute with deep breathing.

7. Loosen the hand grip, straighten the legs and repeat the pose on the other side. Here, bring both the feet beside the left hip, turn the trunk to the right, straighten the left arm, place the left palm underneath the right knee and catch the left upper arm near the elbow with the right hand from behind the back. Stay there for an equal length of time.

Effects

This simple āsana works on the dorsal and lumbar regions of the spine. People with very stiff backs find the other lateral twisting positions extremely difficult. This pose helps to make the back supple. People with arthritis will find it very beneficial.

54. *Marīchyāsana II* Ten* (Plates 135 and 136)

This is one of the sitting lateral twisting postures.

Technique

1. Sit on the floor with the legs stretched straight in front. (Plate 35)

2. Bend the left knee, place the sole and heel of the left foot flat on the floor. The shin of the left leg should be perpendicular to the floor and the calf should touch the thigh. Place the left heel near the perineum. The inner side of the left foot should touch the inner side of the outstretched right thigh.

3. With an exhalation, turn the spine about 90 degrees to the left, so that the chest goes beyond the bent left thigh and bring the right arm over the left thigh. (Plate 133)

4. Place the right shoulder beyond the left knee and stretch the right arm out forwards by turning the spine still more to the left and stretching the region at the back of the right floating ribs. (Plate 134) Take two breaths.

5. With an exhalation, twist the right arm round the left

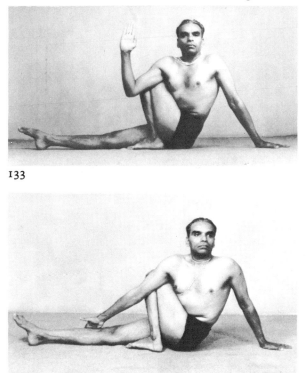

133

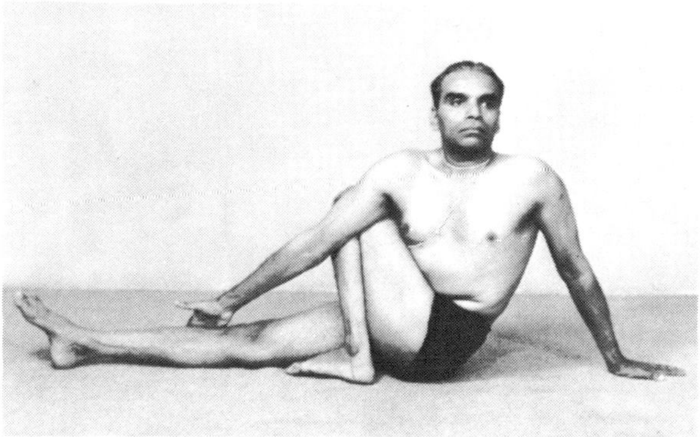

134

knee, flex the right elbow and place the right wrist at the back of the waist. Inhale and hold the pose.

6. Exhale deeply and turn the left arm from the shoulder behind the back. Either clasp the left hand behind the back with the right hand or vice versa. (Plates 135 and 136) In the beginning, one finds it difficult to twist the trunk sideways, but with practice, the armpit touches the bent knee. After one has twisted the arm round the knee, one also finds it difficult to clasp the fingers of one hand with the other.

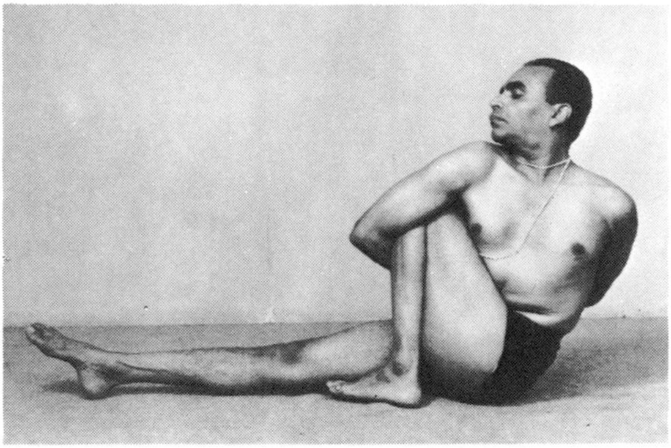

135

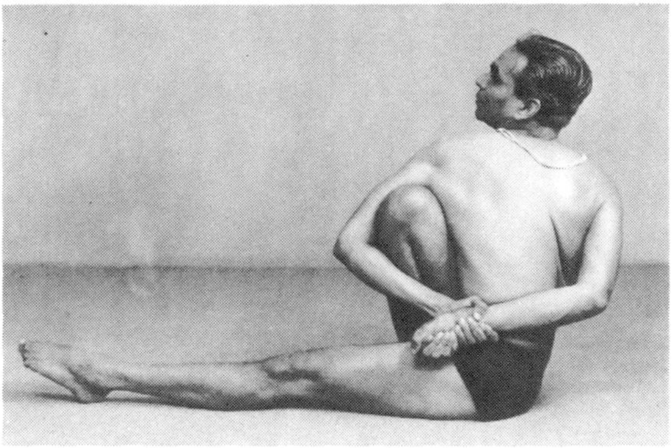

136

Gradually one learns to clasp the fingers, then the palm and lastly to hold the hand at the wrist behind the back.

7. The right arm should lock the left bent knee tightly. There should be no space between the right armpit and the bent left knee.

8. After clasping the hands at the back, turn the spine still more to the left by tugging at the clapsed hands.

9. The whole of the outstretched right leg should remain straight and securely on the floor, but you will not be able to achieve this to start with. Tighten the muscles of the outstretched thigh so that the knee-cap is pulled up towards the thigh and also tighten the muscles of the calf of the outstretched leg. Then the leg will remain firm and extend on the floor.

10. Stay in this position from half a minute to a minute with normal breathing. The neck may be turned either way to gaze at the toes of the extended leg on the floor or to look over the shoulder.

11. Unclasp the hands at the back and turn the trunk back to its original position. Lower the bent leg and extend it fully on the floor.

12. Then repeat the pose on the other side. This time bend the right knee and place the right foot firmly on the floor so that the right heel touches the perineum and the inner side of the right foot touches the outstretched left thigh. Turn the trunk about 90 degrees to the right so that the left armpit touches the bent right knee. With an exhalation, twist the left arm round the right knee and bring the left hand to the back of the waist. Then throw the right arm behind the back from the shoulder and flexing the right elbow, bring the right hand to the left hand and clasp them. Turn still more to the right and gaze at either the toes of the outstretched left leg or over the right shoulder. Stay on this side also for the same length of time. Unclasp the hands, turn the trunk back to normal, stretch the right leg on the floor and relax.

Effects

By the regular practice of this āsana, splitting backaches, lumbago and pains in the hips disappear rapidly. The liver and the spleen are contracted and so are toned and cease to be sluggish. The muscles of the neck gain power. Sprains in the shoulder and displacement of the shoulder joints are relieved and the shoulder movements become free. The intestines also benefit from this āsana. Its effects will be less on lean persons, for whom there are better poses described later. It also helps to reduce the size of the abdomen.

55. *Ardha Matsyendrāsana* Eight* (Plates 139 and 140)
Ardha means half. In the *Haṭha Yoga Pradīpikā*, Matsyendra is mentioned as one of the founders of Haṭha Vidyā. It is related that once Lord Śiva went to a lonely island and explained to his consort Pārvati the mysteries of Yoga. A fish near the shore heard everything with concentration and remained motionless while listening. Śiva, realising that the fish had learnt Yoga, sprinkled water upon it, and immediately the fish gained divine form and became Matsyendra (Lord of the Fishes) and thereafter spread the knowledge of Yoga.

Technique
1. Sit on the floor, with the legs stretched straight in front. (Plate 35)

2. Bend the left knee and join the thigh and calf; raise the seat from the floor, place the left foot under the buttocks and sit on the left foot so that the left heel rests under the left buttock. The foot used as the seat should be kept horizontal on the floor, the outer side of the ankle and the little toe of the foot resting on the ground. If the foot is not so placed, it will be impossible to sit on it. Balance securely in this position.

3. Then bend the right knee and lifting the right leg from the floor, place it by the outer side of the left thigh so that the outer side of the right ankle touches the outer side of the left thigh on the floor. Balance in this position, keeping the right shin perpendicular to the floor. (Plate 137)

4. Turn the trunk 90 degrees to the right until the left armpit touches the outer side of the right thigh. Bring the armpit over the right knee. (Plate 138) Exhale, stretch the left arm from the shoulder and twist it round the right knee. Bend the left elbow and move the left wrist to the back of the waist.

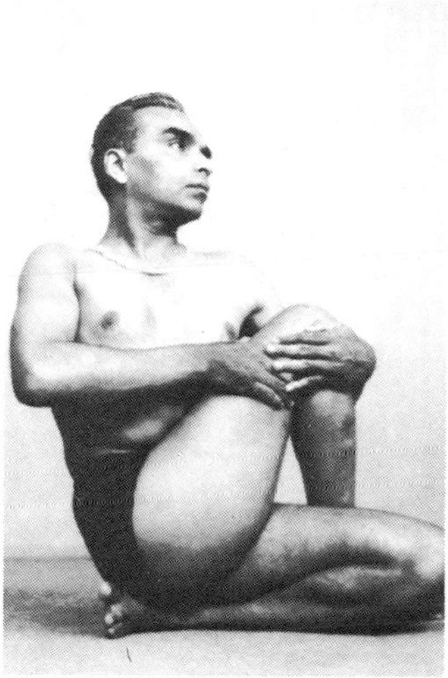

137

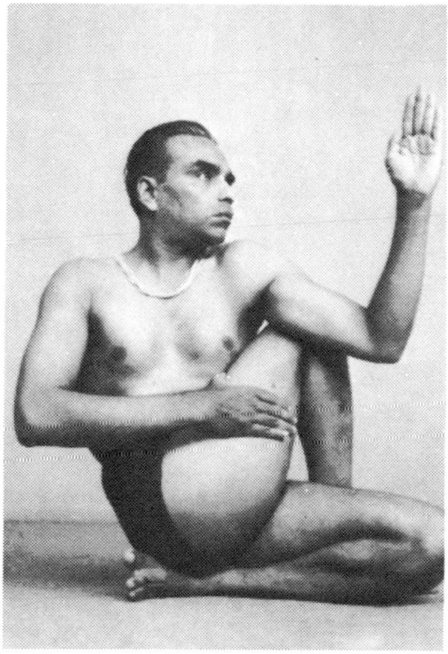

138

5. The left arm should lock the bent right knee tightly and there should be no space between the left armpit and the bent right knee. To achieve this, exhale and move the trunk forward. Stay in this position and take 2 breaths.

6. Now exhale deeply and swing back the right arm from the shoulder, bend the right elbow, move the right hand behind the waist and either clasp it with the left hand or vice versa. At first you will be able to catch a finger or two. With practice it will be possible to catch the palms and then the wrists behind the back.

7. The neck may be turned to the left and the gaze directed over the left shoulder (Plate 139), or to the right, and the gaze fixed at the centre of the eyebrows. (Plate 140) The spinal twist will be greater if the neck is turned to the left than when to the right.

8. As the diaphragm is squeezed by the spinal twist, the breathing will at first become short and fast. Do not be

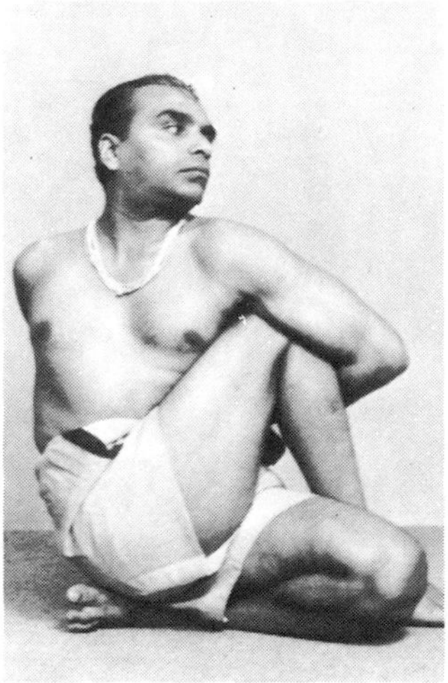

139

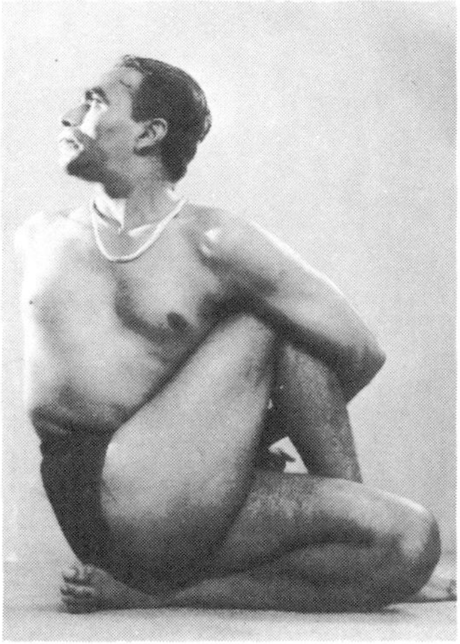

140

nervous. After some practice the pose can be held from half a minute to a minute with normal breathing.

9. Release the hands, remove the right foot from the floor and straighten the right and then the left leg.

10. Repeat the pose on the other side and hold it for the same length of time. Here, bend the right leg and sit on the right foot so that the right heel is under the right buttock. Place the left leg over the right leg and rest the left foot on the floor so that the outer side of the left ankle touches the outer side of the right thigh on the floor. Turn the trunk 90 degrees to the left, placing the right armpit over the left knee and twist the right arm round the left knee. Flex the right elbow and move the right hand behind the waist. Hold the pose and take 2 breaths. Again exhale completely and swing the left arm back from the shoulder, bend the left elbow and clasp the hands behind the back at the wrist. Then release and relax.

11. In the beginning it may not be possible to twist either arm round the opposite knee. In that case try and hold the

opposite foot, keeping the arm straight at the elbow. It also takes time to clasp the hands behind the back. Gradually, the backward stretch of the arms will increase, and one will be able to catch at first the fingers, next the palms, then the wrist and as the pose is mastered even the forearms above the wrists. Beginners who find it difficult to sit on the foot can sit on the floor.

Effects

By the practice of this āsana, one derives the benefits mentioned under Marīchyāsana III. (Posture 54 and Plate 135) But here as the range of movement is more intensified, the effects will also be greater. In Marīchyāsana III the upper part of the abdomen is squeezed. Here the lower part of the abdomen has the benefit of the exercise. The prostate and bladder are not enlarged if one practices regularly.

56. *Ūrdhva Dhanurāsana* Seven* (Plate 144)

Ūrdhva means upwards. Dhanu means a bow. In this posture the body is arched back and supported on the palms and soles.

Technique

1. Lie flat on the back on the floor. (Plate 48)

2. Bend and raise the elbows over the head, and place the palms under the shoulders. The distance between the palms should not be wider than the shoulders and the fingers should point towards the feet.

3. Bend and raise the knees, then bring the feet nearer until they touch the hips. (Plate 141)

4. Exhale, raise the trunk and rest the crown of the head on the floor. (Plate 142) Take two breaths.

5. Now exhale, lift the trunk and head and arch the back so that its weight is taken on the palms and the soles. (Plate 143)

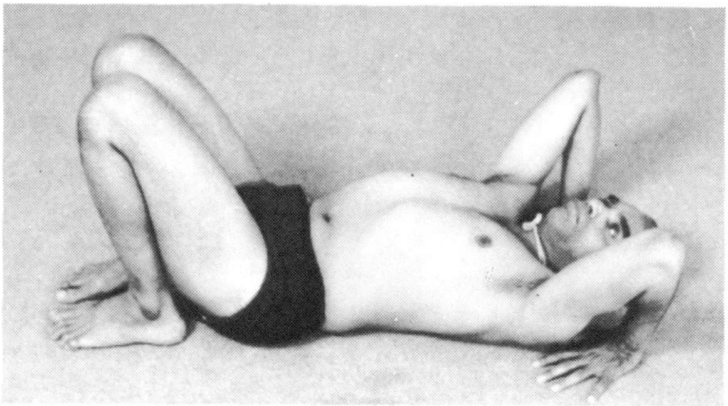

141

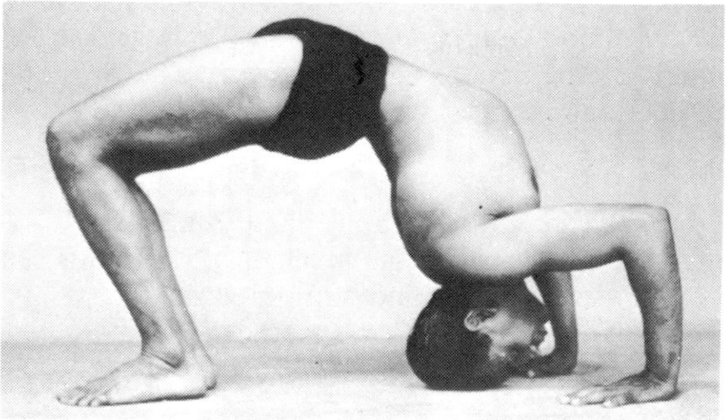

142

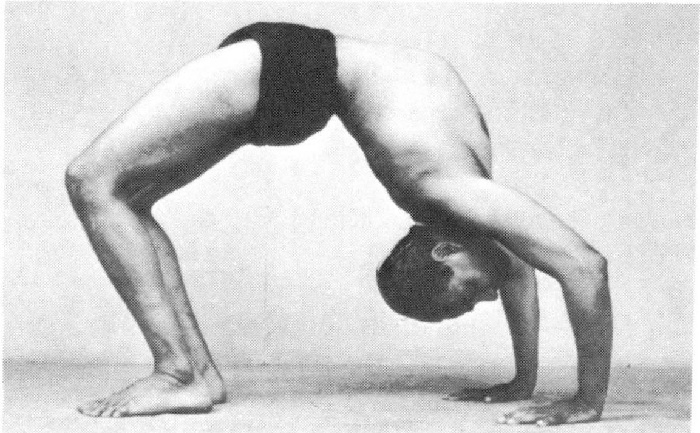

143

6. Stretch the arms from the shoulders until the elbows are straightened, at the same time pulling the thigh muscles up. (Plate 144)

7. To get a better stretch, exhale and pull the thigh muscles still higher by lifting the heels off the floor. (Plate 145). Extend the chest, stretch up the sacral region of the spine until the abdomen is taut as a drum and then lower the heels to the floor, maintaining the stretch of the spine.

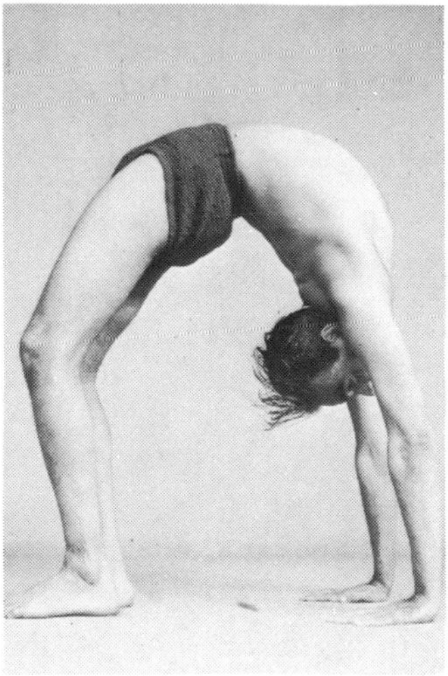
144

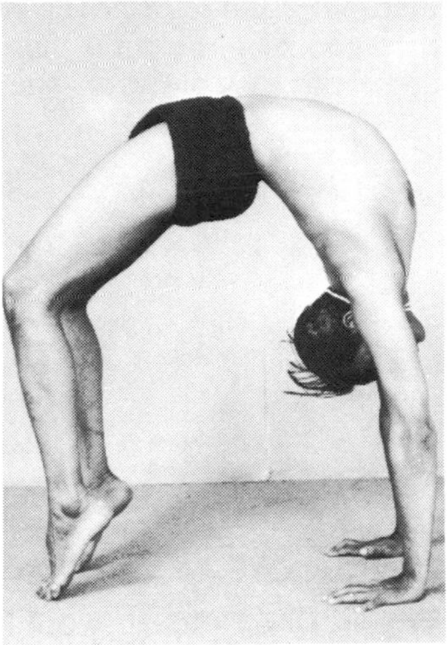
145

8. Remain in this position from half a minute to a minute, with normal breathing.

9. With an exhalation, lower the body to the floor by bending the knees and elbows.

Effects

This āsana is the beginning of the advanced and difficult back-bending poses. It tones the spine by stretching it fully and keeps the body alert and supple. The back feels strong and full of life. It strengthens the arms and wrists and has a very soothing effect on the head. It gives one great vitality, energy and a feeling of lightness.

57. *Śavāsana* (Also called *Mṛtāsana*) (Plate 146)
Śava or Mṛta means a corpse. In this āsana the object is to imitate a corpse. Once life has departed, the body remains still and no movements are possible. By remaining motionless for some time and keeping the mind still while you are fully conscious, you learn to relax. This conscious relaxation invigorates and refreshes both body and mind. But it is much harder to keep the mind than the body still. Therefore, this apparently easy posture is one of the most difficult to master.

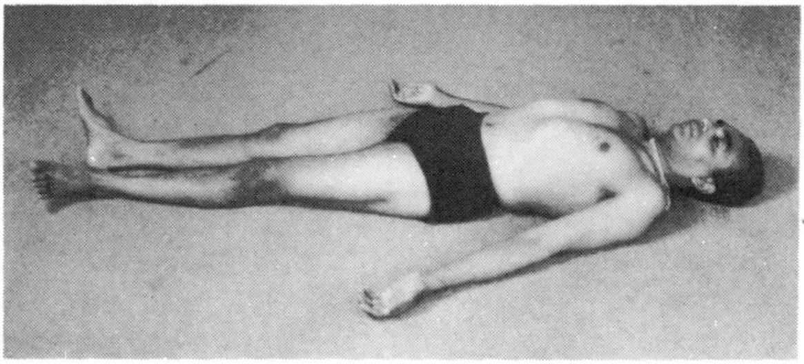

146

Technique

1. Lie flat on the back full length like a corpse. Keep the hands a little away from the thighs, with the palms up.

2. Close the eyes. If possible place a black cloth folded four times over the eyes. Keep the heels together and the toes apart.

3. To start with breathe deeply. Later the breathing should be fine and slow, with no jerky movements to disturb the spine or the body.

4. Concentrate on deep and fine exhalations, in which the nostrils do not feel the warmth of breath.

5. The lower jaw should hang loose and not be clenched. The tongue should not be disturbed, and even the pupils of the eyes should be kept completely passive.

6. Relax completely and breathe out slowly.

7. If the mind wanders, pause without any strain after each slow exhalation.

8. Stay in the pose from 15 to 20 minutes.

9. One is apt to fall asleep in the beginning. Gradually, when the nerves become passive, one feels completely relaxed and refreshed.

When well relaxed one feels energy flow from the back of the head towards the heels and not the other way round. One also feels as if the body is elongated.

Effects

Verse 32 of the First Chapter of the *Haṭha Yoga Pradīpikā* states: 'Lying upon one's back on the ground at full length like a corpse is called Śavāsana. This removes the fatigue caused by the other āsanas and induces calmness of mind.'

Mṛtāsana is thus described in verse 11 of the Second Chapter of the *Gheraṇḍa Saṁhitā*: 'Lying flat on the ground (on one's back) like a corpse is called Mṛtāsana. This posture destroys fatigue, and quiets the agitation of the mind.'

'The mind is the lord of the Indriyas (the organs of senses); the Praṇa (the Breath of Life) is the lord of the mind.' 'When the mind is absorbed it is called Mokṣa (final emancipation, liberation of the soul); when Prāṇa and Manas (the mind) have been absorbed, an undefinable joy ensues.' Verses 29 and 30, chapter IV, *Haṭha Yoga Pradīpikā*.

To tame Prāṇa depends upon the nerves. Steady, smooth, fine and deep breathing without any jerky movements of the body soothes the nerves and calms the mind. The stresses of modern civilisation are a strain on the nerves for which Śavāsana is the best antidote.

Part III

Prāṇāyāma

Hints and Cautions

Read and digest thoroughly the following hints and cautions before attempting the prāṇāyāma techniques mentioned later.

Qualifications for fitness

1. Just as post-graduate training depends upon the ability and discipline acquired in mastering the subject in which one graduated, so prāṇāyāma training demands mastery of āsanas and the strength and discipline arising therefrom.

2. The fitness of the aspirant for training and advancement in Prāṇāyāma is to be gauged by an experienced Guru or teacher and his personal supervision is essential.

3. Pneumatic tools can cut through the hardest rock. In Prāṇāyāma the yogi uses his lungs as pneumatic tools. If they are not used properly, they destroy both the tool and the person using it. The same is true of prāṇāyāma.

Cleanliness and Food

4. One does not enter a temple with a dirty body or mind. Before entering the temple of his own body, the yogi observes the rules of cleanliness.

5. Before starting prāṇāyāma practices the bowels should be evacuated and the bladder emptied. This leads to comfort in the bandhas.

6. Preferably prāṇāyāma should be practised on an empty stomach, but if this is difficult, a cup of milk, tea, coffee or cocoa may be taken. Allow at least six hours to elapse after a meal before practising prāṇāyāma.

7. Light food may be taken half an hour after finishing prāṇāyāma practices.

Time and Place

8. The best time for practice is in the early morning (preferably before sunrise) and after sunset. According to the *Haṭha Yoga Pradīpikā*, prāṇāyāma should be practised four times a day, in the early morning, noon, evening and midnight, with 80 cycles at a time (chapter II, verse 11). This is hardly possible in the fast modern age. What is therefore recommended is to practice at least 15 minutes a day, but the 80 cycles are for intensely devoted practitioners, and not for the average householder.

9. The best seasons in which to start the practice are spring and autumn when the climate is equable.

10. Prāṇāyāma should be done in a clean airy place, free from insects. Since noise creates restlessness practice during quiet hours.

11. Prāṇāyāma should be practised with determination and regularity at the same time and place and in the same posture. Variation is permissible only in the type of prāṇāyāma practised, that is to say, if Sūrya Bhedana Prāṇāyāma is done one day, Śitalī may be done the next day and Bhastrikā be done on the third day. Nāḍī Sodhana Prāṇāyāma, however, should be practised daily.

Posture

12. Breathing in prāṇāyāma practices is done through the nose only, except in Śitalī and Śitakāri.

13. Prāṇāyāma is best done sitting on the floor on a folded blanket. The postures suitable are Siddhāsana, Vīrāsana, Padmāsana and Baddhakoṇāsana. Any other sitting posture may be taken provided the back is kept absolutely erect from the base of the spine to the neck and perpendicular to the floor. Some types, however, may be done in a reclining position as detailed later.

14. During practice no strain should be felt in the facial

muscles, eyes and ears, or in the neck muscles, shoulders, arms, thighs and feet. The thighs and arms should be relaxed deliberately since they are unconsciously tensed during prāṇāyāma.

15. Keep the tongue passive or saliva will accumulate in the mouth. If it does, swallow it before exhalation (rechaka) and not while holding the breath (kumbhaka).

16. During inhalation and retention the rib cage should expand both forwards and sideways, but the area below the shoulder-blades and armpits should only expand forwards.

17. To start with there will be perspiration and trembling which will disappear in course of time.

18. In all the prāṇāyāma practices done in a sitting posture, the head should hang down from the nape of the neck, the chin resting in the notch between the collar-bones on the top of the breast-bone. This chinlock or Jālandhara Bandha should be used except where specifically stated in the techniques hereafter given.

19. Keep the eyes closed throughout as otherwise the mind will wander after outside objects and be distracted. The eyes, if kept open, will feel a burning sensation, and irritability.

20. No pressure should be felt inside the ear during the practice of prāṇāyāma.

21. The left arm is kept straight, the back of the wrist resting on the left knee. The forefinger is bent towards the thumb, its tip touching the tip of the thumb. This is the Jñāna Mudrā described later in the technique.

22. The right arm is bent at the elbow and the hand is kept on the nose to regulate the even flow of breath and to gauge its subtlety. This is felt through the tips of the ring and little fingers which control the left nostril and through the tip of

the thumb which controls the right nostril. Details of the right hand position are discussed in the technique. In some methods of prāṇāyāma both the hands rest on the knees in the Jñāna Mudrā.

23. When a baby learns to walk by itself, the mother remains passive bodily, but alert mentally. In an emergency, as when the child stumbles, her body springs into action to save it from a fall. So also, in the practice of prāṇāyāma the brain is kept passive but alert. Whenever the organs of the body fail to work properly, the watchful brain sends messages of warning. The ear is told to listen for the proper sound of the breath (which is described below). The hand and nose are told to observe the sensitivity of the breath flowing through the nasal passages.

24. It may be asked that if the brain is required to send warnings to the senses, how can one concentrate on prāṇāyāma? A painter absorbed in his work notes various details like perspective and composition, the colour tones and shades, the foreground and background and the strokes of the paint-brush all at once. A musician playing a melody watches his finger movements and sound patterns, the tuning of the instrument and its pitch. Though the artist and the musician are both observing and correcting the details, they are concentrating on their work. So also the yogi observes details like time, posture and an even breath rhythm, and is alert and sensitive to the flow of prāṇa within him.

25. As a careful mother teaches her child to walk carefree, so the careful mind of the yogi teaches the senses to be carefree. By continued practice of prāṇāyāma the senses become free of obsession for the things they once pined for.

26. Each should measure his own capacity when doing prāṇāyāma and not exceed it. This may be gauged as follows: suppose one can with comfort inhale and exhale for 10 seconds each in rhythmic cycles for a given length of time, say 5 minutes. If there is any change in the rhythm in which

the period of inhalation decreases, to say 7 or 8 seconds, one has reached one's capacity. To go beyond this point, strains the lungs unduly and brings in its wake a host of respiratory diseases.

27. Faulty practice puts undue stress on the lungs and diaphragm. The respiratory system suffers and the nervous system is adversely affected. The very foundation of a healthy body and a sound mind is shaken by faulty practice of prāṇāyāma. Forceful and strained inhalation or exhalation is wrong.

28. Evenness of breathing leads to healthy nerves and so to evenness of mind and temper.

29. Āsanas should never be practised immediately after prāṇāyāma. If prāṇāyāma is done first, allow an hour to elapse before starting āsanas, for the nerves which are soothed in prāṇāyāma are liable to be ruffled by the bodily movement of the āsanas.

30. Prāṇāyāma, however, may be done not less than 15 minutes after mild practice of āsanas.

31. Strenuous āsanas cause fatigue. When exhausted do not practise prāṇāyāma in any sitting posture, as the back cannot stay erect, the body trembles and the mind becomes disturbed. Deep breathing as in Ujjāyī done in a reclining position relieves fatigue.

32. When deep, steady and long breathing cannot be maintained rhythmically, stop. Do not proceed further. The rhythm should be gauged from the nasal sound produced in inhalation ('ssssssa' which sounds like a leak in a cycle tube) and exhalation (the aspirate 'huuuuuuuuum' sound). If the volume of the sound is reduced, stop.

33. Try to achieve an even ratio in inhalation (puraka) and exhalation (rechaka). For example, if one is for 5 seconds

during a given continuous cycle, the other should be for the same time.

34. The Ujjāyī and Nāḍī Śodhana types of prāṇāyāma are the most beneficial ones which can be practised by pregnant women, preferably in Baddhakoṇāsana. During pregnancy, however, the breath should never be held without the guidance of an experienced teacher.

35. After completing any prāṇāyāma practice always lie down on the back like a corpse in Śavāsana (Plate 146) for at least 5 or 10 minutes in silence. The mind should be completely switched off and every limb and sense organ completely passive as if dead. Śavāsana after prāṇāyāma refreshes both the body and the mind.

Kumbhakas

36. Thorough mastery of inhalation (puraka) and exhalation (rechaka) is essential before any attempt is made to learn antara kumbhaka (retention following inhalation).

37. Bāhya kumbhaka (restraint following exhalation) should not be tried until antara kumbhaka has become natural.

38. During the practice of kumbhaka there is a tendency to draw in air as well as to tighten and loosen the diaphragm and abdominal organs for the sake of increasing the period of retention. This is unconscious and unintentional. Care should be taken to avoid it.

39. If it is found difficult to hold the breath (khumbaka) after each inhalation or exhalation, do some cycles of deep breathing and then practise kumbhakas. For instance, 3 cycles of deep breathing may be followed by one cycle of kumbhaka. Then there should be another 3 cycles of deep breathing followed by a second cycle of kumbhaka, and so on.

40. If the rhythm of inhalation or exhalation is disturbed by holding the breath, lessen the duration of kumbhaka.

41. Persons suffering from eye or ear trouble (like glaucoma and pus in the ear) should not attempt to hold the breath.

42. Sometimes constipation occurs in the initial stages following upon the introduction of kumbhaka. This is temporary and will disappear in due course.

43. The normal rate of breaths per minute is 15. This rate increases when the body is upset by indigestion, fever, cold and cough, or by emotions like fear, anger or lust. The normal rate of breathing is 21,600 breaths inhaled and exhaled every 24 hours. The yogi measures his span of life not by the number of days, but of breaths. Since breathing is lengthened in prāṇāyāma, its practice leads to longevity.

44. Continuous practice of prāṇāyāma will change the mental outlook of the practitioner and reduce considerably the craving of his senses for worldly pleasures like smoking, drinking and sexual indulgence.

45. In the practice of prāṇāyāma the senses are drawn inwards and in the silence of the kumbhaka the aspirant hears his inner voice calling: 'Look within! The source of all happiness is within!' This also prepares him for the next stage of yoga, pratyāhāra, which leads to freedom from the domination and tyranny of the senses.

46. Since the eyes are kept closed throughout the practice of prāṇāyāma, the passage of time is noted by the mental repetition (japa) of a sacred word or name. This repetition of the sacred words or names is the seed (bīja) planted in the yogi's mind. This seed grows and makes him fit for dhyāna or concentration, the sixth stage of Yoga. Ultimately it produces the fruit of samādhi, where there is experience of full consciousness and supreme joy, where the yogi merges with the Maker of the Universe and feels what he can never express – yet cannot entirely conceal. Words fail to convey the experience adequately, for the mind cannot find words with which to describe it. It is a feeling of that peace which passeth all understanding.

Technique and Effects of Prāṇāyāma

58. *Ujjāyī Prāṇāyāma* (Plate 147)
The prefix ud attached to verbs and nouns, means upwards or superiority in rank. It also means blowing or expanding. It conveys the sense of pre-eminence and power.

Jaya means conquest, victory, triumph or success. Looked at from another viewpoint it implies restraint or curbing.

Ujjāyi is the process in which the lungs are fully expanded and the chest puffed out like that of a proud conqueror.

Technique

1. Sit in any comfortable position like Padmāsana (Plate 53), Siddhāsana (Plate 38) or Vīrāsana (Plate 43).

2. Keep the back erect and rigid. Lower the head to the trunk. Rest the chin in the notch between the collar-bones just above the breast-bone. (This is the Jālandhara Bandha. Jāla means a net, web, lattice or a mesh.)

3. Stretch the arms out straight and rest the back of the wrists on the knees. Join the tips of the index fingers to the tips of the thumbs, keeping the other fingers extended. (This position or gesture of the hand is known as the Jñāna Mudrā, the symbol or seal of knowledge. The index finger symbolises the individual soul and the thumb the Universal Soul. The union of the two symbolises knowledge.)

4. Close the eyes and look inwards. (Plate 147)

5. Exhale completely.

6. Now the Ujjāyi method of breathing begins.

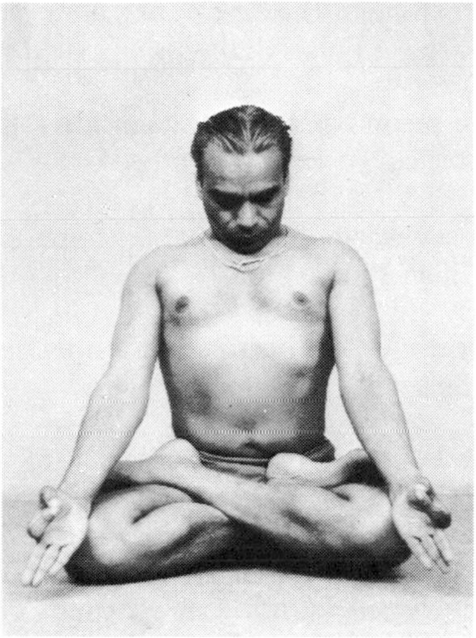

147

7. Take a slow, deep steady breath through both nostrils. The passage of the incoming air is felt on the roof of the palate and makes a sibilant sound (sa). This sound should be heard.

8. Fill the lungs up to the brim. Care should be taken not to bloat the abdomen in the process of inhalation. (Observe this in all types of Prāṇāyāma.) This filling up is called puraka (inhalation).

9. The entire abdominal area from the pubes up to the breat-bone should be pulled back towards the spine.

10. Hold the breath for a second or two.

11. Exhale slowly, deeply and steadily, until the lungs are completely empty. As you begin to exhale, keep your grip on the abdomen. After two or three seconds of exhalation, relax the diaphragm gradually and slowly. While exhaling the passage of the outgoing air should be felt on the roof of the

palate. The brushing of the air on the palate should make an aspirate sound (ha). This exhalation is called rechaka.

12. Wait for a second before drawing a fresh breath. This waiting period is called bāhya kumbhaka.

13. The process described from para. 7 to para. 12 completes one cycle of Ujjāyi Prāṇāyāma.

14. Repeat the cycles for five to ten minutes keeping the eyes closed throughout.

15. Lie on the floor in Śāvāsana. (Plate 146)

16. Ujjāyi Prāṇāyāma may be done without the Jālandhara Bandha even while walking or lying down. This is the only prāṇāyāma which can be done at all times of the day and night.

Effects

This type of prāṇāyāma aerates the lungs, removes phlegm, gives endurance, soothes the nerves and tones the entire system. Ujjāyi without kumbhaka, done in a reclining position, is ideal for persons suffering from high blood pressure or coronary troubles.

59. *Sūrya Bhedana Prāṇāyāma* (Plate 149)

Sūrya is the sun. Bhedana is derived from the root bhid meaning to pierce, to break or pass through.

In Sūrya Bhedana Prāṇāyāma, the breath is inhaled through the right nostril. In other words the prāṇa passes through the Piṅgalā or Sūrya nādī. A kumbhaka is then performed and the breath is then exhaled through the left nostril which is the path of the Idā nāḍī.

Technique

1. Sit in any comfortable position like Padmāsana (Plate 53), Siddhāsana (Plate 38) or Vīrāsana (Plate 43).

2. Keep the back erect and rigid. Lower the head to the trunk. Rest the chin in the notch between the collar-bones just above the breast-bone. (This is Jālandhara Bandha.)

3. Stretch the left arm. Rest the back of the left wrist on the left knee. Perform Jñāna with the left hand (as stated in stage 3 of the technique of Ujjāyi).

4. Bend the right arm at the elbow. Bend the index and middle fingers towards the palm, keeping them passive. Bring the ring and little fingers towards the thumb. (Plate 148)

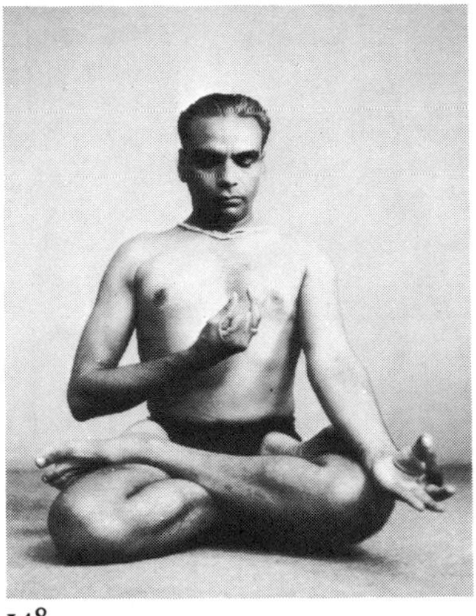

148

5. Place the right thumb on the right side of the nose just below the nasal bone, the ring and little fingers on the left side of the nose just below the nasal bone, just above the curve of the fatty tissue of the nostrils above the upper jaw.

6. Press the ring and the little finger to block the left side of the nose completely.

7. With the right thumb, press the fatty tissue on the right side so as to make the outer edge of the right nostril parallel to the lower edge of the cartilage of the septum.

8. The right thumb is bent at the top joint and the tip of the thumb is placed at a right angle to the septum. (Plate 149)

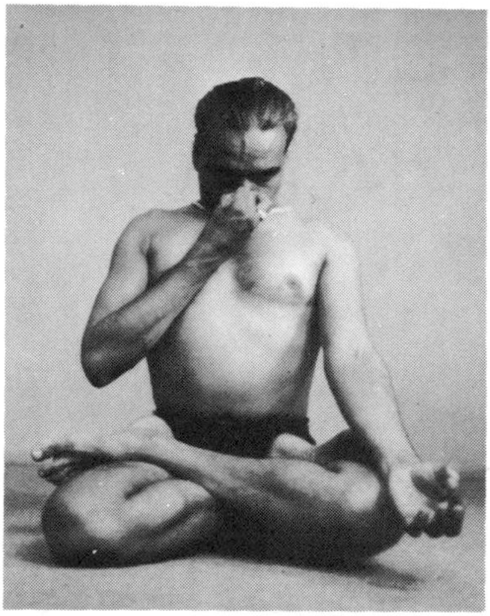

149

9. Now inhale slowly and deeply controlling the aperture of the right nostril with the tip of the thumb nearer the nail. Fill the lungs to the brim (puraka).

10. Then block the right nostril so that both are now blocked.

11. Hold the breath for about 5 seconds (antara kumbhaka)

12. Keeping the right nostril completely blocked, open the left nostril partially and exhale through it slowly and deeply (rechaka).

13. During the exhalation regulate the rhythmic flow of air

from the left nostril by adjusting pressure with the ring and little fingers, so that the outer edge of the left notril is kept parallel to the septum. The pressure should be exerted from the inner sides of the tips of the fingers (away from the nails).

14. This completes one cycle of Sūrya Bhedana Prāṇāyāma. Continue with more cycles at a stretch from 5 to 10 minutes, according to capacity.

15. All the inhalations in Sūrya Bhedana are from the right nostril and all the exhalations from the left nostril.

16. Throughout the process, the passage of air is felt at the tips of the fingers and the thumbs and in the nasal membranes where pressure is applied. The passage of air makes a sound similar to air escaping from a cycle tube. This sound should be maintained constant throughout by varying pressure on the nostrils.

17. The eyes, temples, eyebrows and the skin on the forehead should remain completely passive and show no sign of strain.

18. The mind should be absorbed completely in listening to the proper sound of the passage of air and in maintaining a proper rhythm in breathing.

19. Each inhalation and exhalation should last for the same length of time.

20. The inhalation and the exhalation should not be forced. An even and slow rhythm should be maintained throughout.

21. Lie down in Śavāsana after completing prāṇāyāma. (Plate 146)

Effects

By reason of the pressure on the nostrils, in this Prāṇāyāma the lungs have to work more than in the case of Ujjāyi. In

Sūrya Bhedana they are filled more slowly, steadily, and fuller than in Ujjāyi. Sūrya Bhedana increases digestive power, soothes and invigorates the nerves, and cleans the sinuses.

Note. It often happens that the passages of both the nostrils are not of the same width, one being bigger than the other. In that case the pressure of the fingers has to be adjusted. In some cases the right nostril is completely blocked while the left one is clear. In that case, inhalation may be done only through the left nostril, while exhalation is done only through the right nostril. In course of time due to the manipulation of the fingers the right nostril clears and inhalation through it becomes possible.

Caution. Persons suffering from low blood pressure will derive benefit but those with high blood pressure or heart trouble should not hold their breath after inhalation (antara kumbhaka) whilst practising this prāṇāyāma.

60. *Nāḍī Śodhana Prāṇāyāma*

Nāḍī is a tubular organ of the body like an artery or a vein for the passage of prāṇa or energy. A nāḍī has three layers like an insulated electric wire. The innermost layer is called sirā, the middle layer damanī and the entire organ as well as the outer layer is called nāḍī.

Śodhana meaning purifying or cleansing, so the object of Nāḍī Śodhana Prāṇāyāma is the purification of the nerves. A little obstruction in a water pipe can cut off the supply completely. A little obstruction in the nerves can cause great discomfort and paralyse a limb or organ.

Technique

1. Follow the technique given in paras 1 to 8 of Sūrya Bhedana Prāṇāyāma. (Plate 149)

2. Empty the lungs completely through the right nostril. Control the aperture of the right nostril with the inner side of the right thumb, away from the nail.

3. Now inhale slowly, steadily and deeply through the right nostril, controlling the aperture with the tip of the right thumb near the nail. Fill the lungs to the brim (puraka). During this inhalation the left nostril is completely blocked by the ring and little fingers.

4. After full inhalation, block the right nostril completely with the pressure of the thumb and release the pressure of the ring and little fingers on the left nostril. Readjust them on the outer edge of the left nostril and keep it parallel to the septum. Exhale slowly, steadily and deeply through the left nostril. Empty the lungs completely. The pressure should be exerted from the inner sides of the tips of the ring and little fingers (away from the nails) (rechaka).

5. After full exhalation through the left nostril, change the pressure on it by adjusting the fingers. In the changed position, the tips of the ring and little fingers nearer the nails exert the pressure.

6. Now inhale through the left nostril slowly, steadily and deeply, filling the lungs to the brim (puraka).

7. After full inhalation through the left nostril, block it and exhale through the right nostril, adjusting the pressure of the right thumb on the right nostril as stated in para. 2 above (rechaka).

8. This completes one cycle of Nāḍī Śodhana Prāṇāyāma. Here the rhythm of breathing is as follows:

(a) Exhale through the right nostril.
(b) Inhale through the right nostril.
(c) Exhale through the left nostril.
(d) Inhale through the left nostril.
(e) Exhale through the right nostril.
(f) Inhale through the right nostril.
(g) Exhale through the left nostril.
(h) Inhale through the left nostril.
(i) Exhale through the right nostril.

(j) Inhale through the right nostril . . . and so on.

Stage (a) above is the preparatory one. The first real Nāḍī Śodhana Prāṇāyāma cycle starts at stage (b) and ends at stage (e). The second cycle starts at stage (f) and ends at stage (i). Stage (j) is the safety measure to be observed after the completion of the cycles in order to prevent gasping, breathlessness and strain on the heart.

9. Do 8 to 10 cycles at a stretch as described above. This may take 6 or 8 minutes.

10. Inhalation and exhalation from each side should take the same time. In the beginning the duration will be unequal. Persevere until equality is achieved.

11. After achieving mastery over the equal duration and precision over inhalation and exhalation on either side an attempt may be made to retain breath (antara kumbhaka) after inhaling.

12. This precision is only achieved after long practice.

13. Retention should not disturb the rhthym and equality of inhalation and exhalation. If either are disturbed curtail the period of retention or hold the breath on alternate cycles.

14. Do not attempt to hold the breath after exhalation (bāhya kumbhaka) until you have mastered retention after inhalation (antara kumbhaka).

15. Retention and the lengthening of inhalation and exhalation should only be attempted with the help and under the guidance of an experienced Guru.

16. Always conclude by lying down in Śavāsana. (Plate 146)

Effects

The blood receives a larger supply of oxygen in Nāḍī Śodhana than in normal breathing, so that one feels refreshed and the nerves are calmed and purified. The mind becomes still and lucid.

Note. In the beginning the body perspires and shakes, while the thigh and arm muscles become tense. Such tension should be avoided.

Caution

1. Persons suffering from high blood pressure or heart trouble should never attempt to hold their breath (kumbhaka). They can practise Nāḍī Śodhana Prāṇāyāma without retention (kumbhaka) with beneficial effect.

2. Persons suffering from low blood pressure can do this prāṇāyāma with retention after inhalation (antara kumbhaka) *only,* with beneficial effects.

61. *Viloma Prāṇāyāma*

Loma means hair. The particle vi is used to denote negation or privation. Viloma thus means against the hair, against the grain, against the natural order of things.

In Viloma Prāṇāyāma inhalation or exhalation is not one uninterrupted continuous process, but is interrupted by several pauses. For instance, if continuous inhalation to fill the lungs or continuous exhalation to expel the air were to take 15 seconds in each case, in Viloma there would be a pause of about 2 seconds after every third second of inhalation or of exhalation. The process of inhalation or of exhalation is thus lengthened to 25 seconds. The technique given below is in two stages, which are distinct.

Technique: Stage I

1. Viloma Prāṇāyāma can be done either in a sitting posture or while lying down.

2. If done when seated, keep the back erect, lower the head to the trunk so that the chin rests in the notch between the collar-bones on the top of the breast-bone. This is Jālandhara

Bandha. Keep the hands in Jñāna Mundra (see p. 189, para 21).

3. Inhale for 2 seconds, pause for 2 seconds holding the breath, again inhale for 2 seconds, again pause for 2 seconds holding the breath, and continue like this until the lungs are completely full.

4. Now hold the breath for 5 to 10 seconds (antara kumbhaka) according to capacity.

5 Exhale slowly and deeply as in Ujjāyi with an aspirate sound (huuuum).

6. This completes one cycle of the first stage of Viloma Prāṇāyāma.

7. Repeat 10 to 15 cycles of this first stage at a stretch.

Stage II

8. Rest for a minute or two.

9. Then take a deep breath without any pauses as in Ujjāyi with a sibilant sound (sssssssa), keeping the chin on the top of the breastbone. Fill the lungs completely.

10. Hold the breath from 5 to 10 seconds (antara kumbhaka), keeping the Mūla Bandha grip.

11. Exhale for 2 seconds and pause for 2 seconds. Again exhale for 2 seconds, pause for 2 seconds and continue like this until the lungs are completely emptied.

12. This completes one cycle of the second stage of Viloma Prāṇāyāma.

13. Repeat the second stage of Viloma 10 to 15 times at a stretch.

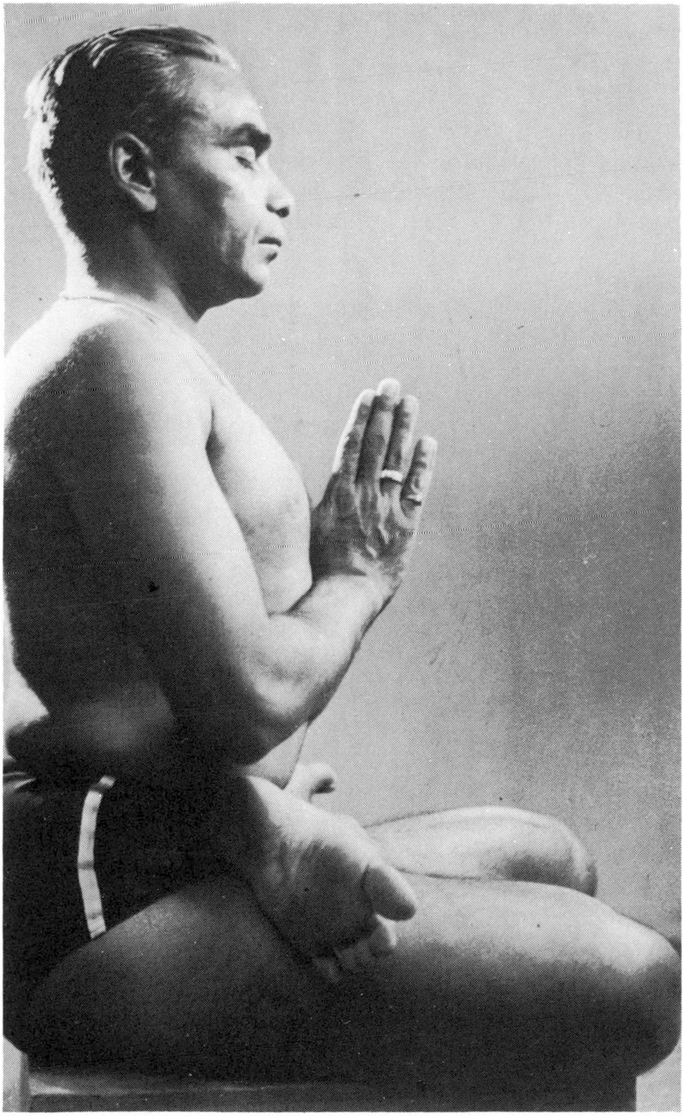

150

14. This completes Viloma Prāṇāyāma.

15. Then lie down in Śavāsana. (Plate 146)

Effects

Viloma Prāṇāyāma in the first stage helps those suffering from low blood pressure. In the second stage it benefits persons suffering from high blood pressure.

Caution

1. The second stage of Viloma should only be done when lying down by persons suffering from high blood pressure.

2. Those suffering from heart complaints should not attempt it until they have mastered the Nāḍī Śodhana and Ujjāyi Prāṇāyāmas.

As a wind drives smoke and impurities from the atmosphere, prāṇāyāma drives away the impurities of the body and the mind. Then, says Patañjali, the DIVINE FIRE within blazes forth in its full glory and the mind becomes fit for concentration (dhāraṇā) and meditation (dhyāna). (*Yoga Sutras,* chapter II, 52 and 53.) This takes a long time. By degrees is the darkness banished by the dawn.

Appendix

Āsana Courses

I am giving the āsanas in a serial order for practice and the possible time it may take to gain control of them.

(The figures within the brackets after the āsanās denote the serial number of the illustrations.)

1st and 2nd week
Tādāsana (1); Utthita Trikoṇāsana (3 and 4); Utthita Pārśvakoṇāsana (5 and 6); Sālamba Sarvāngāsana (102); Halāsana (113); Savāsana (146).

3rd and 4th week
Utthita Trikoṇāsana (3 and 4); Utthita Pārśvakoṇāsana (5 and 6); Vīrabhadrāsana I & II (9 and 10); Pārśvottānāsana (13); Sālamba Sarvāngāsana (102); Halāsana (115); Śavāsana (146).

5th and 6th week
Utthita Trikoṇāsana (3 and 4); Utthita Pārśvakoṇāsana (5 and 6); Vīrabhadrāsana I and II (9 and 10); Pārśvottānāsana (13); Prasārita Pādottānāsana (17); Stay ½ a minute on each side in all these āsanās. Paripūrna Nāvāsana (36); Sālamba Sarvāngāsana (102); Halāsana (113); Paschimottānāsana (81); Śavāsana (146).

7th and 8th week
Utthita Trikoṇāsana (3 and 4); Utthita Pārśvakoṇāsana (5 and 6); Vīrabhadrāsana I and II (9 and 10); Pārśvottānāsana (13); Prasārita Pādottānāsana (17); Pādānguṣṭhāsana (22); Pāda Hastāsana (24); Uttānāsana (25); Sālamba Sarvāngāsana (102); Halāsana (113); Karṇapīdāsana (114); Danḍāsana (35); Paripurṇa Nāvāsana (36); Ardha Nāvāsana (37); Paschimottānāsana (81); Poorvottānāsana (82); Śavāsana (146).

9th week
Consolidate the āsanās and increase the length of stay in all of them.

10th week
Repeat all the āsanās and do Ujjāyī Prāṇāyāma (Section 58) without sitting in Siddhāsana (38) for 5 minutes and do Śavāsana (146) for 5 minutes.

11th and 12th week
Utthita Trikoṇāsana (3 and 4); Utthita Pārśvakoṇāsana (5 and 6); Vīrabhadrāsana I and II (9 and 10); Pārśvottānāsana (13); Prasārita Pādottānāsana (17) Pādānguṣṭhāsana (22); Pāda Hastāsana (24); Uttānāsana (25); Danḍāsana (35); Paripūrna Nāvāsana (36); Ardha Nāvāsana (37); Mahā Mudrā (61); Jānu Śīrsāsana (63); Paschimottānāsana (81); Poorvottānāsana (82); Chaturanga Danḍāsana (30) Bhujangāsana (31); Śalabhāsana (26); Dhanurāsana (28) Urdhva Mukha-Śvānāsana (32); Uṣṭrāsana (20); Adho Mukha Śvānāsana (33); Baddha Koṇāsana (51); Sālamba Sarvāngāsana (102); Halāsana (113); Karṇapīdāsana (114); Supta Koṇāsana (115); Pārśva Halāsana (116); Śavāsana (146) for 5 minutes; Ujjāyī Prāṇāyāma without retention (Section 58) in Siddhāsana (38) for 5 minutes.

13th week
Repeat. Do Ujjāyī Prāṇāyāma with inhalation retention (Section 58) in Siddhāsāna (38) or in Śavāsana (146).

14th to 18th week (Observe the change in the order of the āsanās)
Sālamba Śīrṣāsana (90); Utthita Trikoṇāsana (3 and 4); Utthita Pārśvakoṇāsana (5 and 6); Vīrabhadrāsana I and II (9 and 10); Pārśvottānasana (13); Prasārita Pādottānāsana (17); Pādānguṣṭhāsana (22); Pāda Hastāsana (24); Uttānāsana (25); Mahā Mudrā (61); Jānu Śīrṣāsana (63); Ardha Baddha Padma Paschimottānāsana (66) Paschimottānāsana (81); Paripoorṇa Nāvāsana (36); Ardha Nāvāsana (37); Pūrvottanāsāna (82); Uṣṭrāsana (20); Śalabhāsana (26);

Dhanurāsana (28) Chaturanga Dandāsana (30); Bhujangāsana (31); Ūrdha Mukha Śvānāsana (32); Adho Mukha Śvānāsana (33); Virāsana (42); Baddha Koṇāsana (51); Sālamba Sarvāngāsana (102); Halāsana (113); Karṇapīdāsana (114); Supta Koṇāsana (115); Pārśva Halāsana (116); Eka Pāda Sarvāngāsana (117); Pārśvaika Pāda Sarvāngāsana (118); Jaṭara Parivartanāsana (127 and 128); Śavāsana (146). Do Ujjāyī Prāṇāyāma (without inhalation retention) (Section 58) in Siddhāsana (38) or in Vīrāsana (42) or in Baddhakoṇāsana (50).

19th and 20th week

Repeat.

If you now find all the standing āsanās are easy enough, you can do them on alternate days or twice a week. The day you do not do the standing āsanās, devote your time to Ujjāyī Prānāyāma (Section 58) first without inhalation retention for 5 minutes and then with inhalation retention for 5 minutes and then with inhalation retention for 5 minutes.

21st and 23rd week

Sālamba Śīrṣāsana (90); if possible Ūrdhva Danḍāsana (94); Sālamba Sarvāngāsana (102); Halāsana (113); Karṇapīdāsana (114); Supta Koṇāsana (115); Pārśva Halāsana (116); Ekapāda Sarvangāsana (117); Pārśvaika Pāda Sarvangāsana (118); Supta Pādānguṣṭhāsana (130); Jaṭara Parivartanāsana (127 and 128); Jānu Śīrṣāsana (63); Ardha Baddha Padma Paschimottānāsana (66); Triang Mukhaika-pāda Paschimottānāsana (69); Marichyāsana I (71); Paschimottānāsana (81); Upaviṣṭha Koṇāsana (74); Baddhakoṇāsana (51); Pūrvottānāsana (82); Bharadwājāsana (131 and 132); Virāsana (42); Chaturangadanḍāsana (30); Bhujangāsana (31); Ūrdhva Mukha Śvānāsana (32); Adho Mukha Śvānāsana (33); Śalabhāsana (26); Dhanurāsana (28); Uśṭrāsana (20); Uttānāsana (25); Śavāsana (146); Ūjjāyī Prānāyāma (Section 58) without inhalation retention in Śavāsana for 5 minutes and with inhalation retention in Siddhāsana (38); or in Padmāsana (53); or in Vīrāsana (42) or in Baddha Koṇāsana (52).

23rd to 25th week

Follow the serial order up to Padmāsana (53) as in the 21st week. Then Parvatāsana (54); Matsyāsana (56); Vīrāsana (42); Supta Vīrāsana (49); Bharadwājāsana (131 and 132); Marichyāsana II (135 and 136); Poorvottānāsana (82); Chaturanga Daṇḍāsana (30); Urdva Mukha Śvānāsana (32); Adho Mukha Śvānāsana (33); Salabhāsana (26); Dhanurāsana (28); Uṣṭrāsana (20); Ūrdhva Dhanurāsana (144); Śavāsana (146); then do Viloma Prāṇāyāma (Section 61) Stage I for 5 minutes and stage II for 5 minutes in Siddhāsana (38) or Padmāsana (53).

When you do the standing positions, eliminate the various movements of Sarvāngāsana cycle and do the rest. For some it is easy to get Padmāsana earlier than the stipulated period and for some it may take a little longer time to get mastery in the position.

26th to 30th week

Sālamba Śīrṣāsana (90); Ūrdhva Daṇḍāsana (94); Sālamba Sarvāngāsana (102); Halāsana (113); Karṇapīḍāsana (114); Supta Koṇāsana (115); Pārśva Halāsana (116); Eka Pāda Sarvāngāsana (117); Pārśvaikapāda Sarvāngāsana (118); Ūrdva Padmāsana in Sarvāngāsana (122); Piṇḍāsana in Sarvāngāsana (123); Setu Bandha Sarvāngāsana (121); Jaṭara Parivartanāsana (127 and 128); Paripūrṇa Nāvāsana (36); Ardha Nāvāsana (37); Jānu Śīrṣāsana (63); Ardha Baddha Padma Paschimottānāsana (66); Triang Mikhaika Pāda Paschimottānāsana (69); Marichyāsana I (71); Paschimottānāsana (81); Upaviṣṭha Koṇāsana (74); Baddha Koṇāsana (51); Padmāsana (53); Parvatāsana (54); Baddha Padmāsana (58 and 59); Yoga Mudrāsana (60); Matyāsana (56); Vīrāsana (42); Supta Vīrāsana (49); Bharadwājāsana (131 and 132); Marichyāsana II (135 and 136); Ardha Matsyendrāsana (139 and 140); Adho Mukha Śvānāsana (33); Ūrdhva Mukha Śvānāsana (32); Chaturanga Daṇḍāsana (30); Śalabhāsana (26); Dhanurāsana (28); Bhujangāsana (31); Poorvottānāsana (82); Uṣṭrāsana (20); Ūrdhva Dhanurāsana (144) for 4 times; Śavāsana (146). Ujjāyī Prāṇāyāma with Antar Kumbhaka (inhalation retention Section 58) and Viloma

Prāṇāyāma (Section 61) in Siddhāsana (38); or in Vīrāsana (42) or in Padmāsana (53).

31st to 32nd week

Consolidate all the āsanās concentrating on perfection as well as timings. Stay in all the forward bendings for a minute on each āsanā and Paschimottānāsana for 5 minutes.

32nd to 35th week

Follow the serial order up to Pinḍāsana in Sarvāngāsana (123) as in the 26th week. Then Pārśva Pinḍāsana in Sarvāngāsana (124 and 125) and continue the serial order from Setu Bandha Sarvāngāsana (121) as in the 26th week up to Śavāsana (146). Do Sūrya Bhedana Prāṇāyāma for 5 minutes and Nāḍi Śodhaṇa Prāṇāyāma 8 cycle only without retention. Sit in Dhyāna (Plate 150) for 3 to 5 minutes.

The following is a course which covers one week and will benefit the body and bring harmony to the mind.

First day of the week

Sālamba Śīrṣāsana (90) for 10 minutes; Ūrdhva Danḍāsana (94) for 1 minute; Sālamba Sarvāngāsana (10 minutes; Halāsana (113) for 5 minutes; Utthita Trikoṇāsana (3 and 4) for 30 seconds on each side; Utthita Pārśva Konāsana (5 and 6) for 30 seconds on each side; Virabhadrāsana I and II for 20 seconds on each side; Pārśvottānāsana (13) for 1 minute on each side; Prasārita Padottānāsana (17) for 1 minute; Pādānguṣṭāsana (22) for 30 seconds; Pāda Hastāsana (24) for 30 seconds; Uttānāsana (25) for 1 minute; Paschimottānāsana (81) for 5 minutes; Poorvottānāsana (82) for 30 seconds; Marīchyāsana II (135 and 136) for 30 seconds on each side; Ardha Matsyendrāsana (139 and 140) for 30 seconds on each side; Ūrdhva Dhanurāsana for 8 to 10 times staying 15 seconds each time; Śavāsana (146) for 5 minutes. Ūjjāyi Prāṇāyāma (with inhalation retention) (Section 58) for 15 minutes and meditation (150) to the capacity, in any āsana. Again Śavāsana (146) for 5 minutes.

Second day of the week

Sālamba Śīrṣāsana (90) for 10 minutes; Ūrdhva Daṇḍāsana (94) from 30 seconds to 1 minute; Sālamba Sarvāngāsana (102) for 10 minutes; Halāsana (113) for 5 minutes; Jaṭara Parivartanāsana (127) for half a minute on each side; Supta Pādānguṣṭāsana (130) for 20 seconds on each side; Paripūrṇa Nāvāsana (36) for 1 minute; Ardha Nāvāsana (37) 20 to 30 seconds; Paschimottānāsana (81) for 5 minutes; Bharadwājāsana (131 and 132) for 30 seconds each side; Marīchyāsana II (135 and 136) for 30 seconds each side; Ardha Matyendrāsana (139 and 140) for 30 seconds on each side; Parvātāsana (54) for 1 minute; Vīrāsana (42) for 1 minute; Supta Vīrāsana (49) for 1 minute; Uṣṭrāsana (20) for 30 seconds; Śalabhāsana (26) for 20 to 30 seconds; Dhanurāsana (28) for 30 seconds; Ūrdhva Mukha Śvānāsana (32) for 20 to 30 seconds; Adho Mukha Śvāṇāsana (33) for 1 minute; Uttānāsana (25) for 1 to 2 minutes; Śavāsana (146) for 5 minutes and Sūrya Bhedana Prāṇāyāma (Section 59) in Padmāsana (53) or in Siddhāsana (38) or in Vīrāsana (42) for 5 minutes and Nādi Śodhana Prāṇāyāma without retention for 10 minutes and sit in Dhyāna (150) for 2 minutes. Again do Śavāsana (146) for 5 minutes.

Third day of the week

Sālamba Śīrṣāsana (90) for 10 minutes, Ūrdhva Daṇḍāsana (94) for 1 minute; Sālamba Sarvāngāsana (102) for 10 minutes; Halāsana (113) for 5 minutes; Karṇapīdāsana (114) for 30 seconds; Supta Koṇāsana (115) for 30 seconds; Pārśva Halāsana (116) for 30 seconds on each side; Eka Pāda Sarvāngāsana (117) for 30 seconds on each side; Pārśvaikapada Sarvāṇgāsana (118) for 30 seconds on each side; Setu Bandha Sarvāngāsana (121) from 30 seconds to 2 minutes; Ūrdhva Padmāsana in Sarvāngāsana (122) for 30 seconds; Pinḍāsana in Sarvāngāsana (123) for 30 seconds; Pārśva Pinḍāsana in Sarvāngāsana (124) for 30 seconds on each side; Jaṭara Parivartanāsana (127 and 128) for 30 seconds on each side twice; Supta Pādānguṣṭhāsana (130) for 30 seconds on each side; Marīchyāsana II (135 and 136) from 30 seconds to 60 seconds on each side; Ardha Matsyendrāsana (139 and 140) from 30 seconds to 60 seconds on each side; Paschimottānāsana (81) for 5 minutes; Śavāsana (146) for 5 minutes. Nādiśodhana Prāṇāyāma (Section 60) without Kumbhaka or retention 10 minutes, Sūrya Bhedana Prāṇāyāma (Section 59) 10 cycles; Dhyāna (150) for 5 minutes.

Fourth day of the week
Sālamba Śīrṣāsana (90) for 5 minutes; Ūrdhva Daṇḍāsana (94) for 1 minute; Sālamba Sarvāngāsana (102) for 5 minutes; Halāsana (113) for 5 minutes; Mahā Mudra (61) for 30 seconds on each side; Jānu Śīrṣāsana (63) for 1 minute on each side; Ardha Baddha Padma Paschimottānāsana (66 and 67) for 1 minute on each side; Trianga Mukhaika Pāda Paschimottānāsana (69) for 1 minute on each side; Marīchyāsana I (71) for 1 minute on each side; Upaviṣṭha Koṇāsana (74) for 1 minute; Vīrāsana (42) for 1 minute; Supta Vīrāsana for 1 minute; Baddha Padmāsana (58 and 59) for 1 minute; Yoga Mudrāsana (60) for 1 minute; Parvatāsana (54) for 30 seconds; Baddha Koṇāsana (51) for 1 minute; Paschimottānāsana (81) for 5 minutes; Ujjāyi Prāṇāyāma (Section 58) with inhalation retention to capacity for 8 times. Śavāsana (146) with Viloma Prāṇāyāma (Section 61) Stage I for 5 minutes.

Fifth day of the week
Sālamba Śīrṣāsana (90) for 10 minutes; Ūrdhva Daṇḍāsana (94) for 1 minute; Sālamba Sarvāngāsana (102) for 10 minutes; Halāsana (113) for 5 minutes; Paschimottānāsana (81) for 5 minutes; Bharadwājāsana (131 and 132) for 30 seconds on each side; Marīchyāsana II (135 and 136) for 30 seconds on each side; Ardha Matsyendrāsana (139 and 140) for 30 seconds on each side; Baddha Padmāsana (58 and 59) for 1 minute; Matsyāsana (56) for 30 seconds; Supta Vīrāsana (49) for 1 minute; Śalabhāsana (26) three times of 15 seconds duration; Dhanurāsana (28) for 20 seconds; Bhujangāsana (31) for 30 seconds; Ūrdhva Mukha Śvānāsana (32) for 30 seconds; Ūrdhva Dhanurāsana (144) for 15 times staying to capacity; Śavāsana (146) with Viloma Prāṇāyāma (Section 61) Stage I and Stage II for 5 minutes each. Dhyāna (150) for 5 minutes.

Sixth day of the week

Sālamba Śīrṣāsana (90) for 5 minutes; Utthita Trikoṇāsana (3 and 4) for 15 seconds on each side; Utthita Parśvakoṇāsana (5 and 6) for 15 seconds on each side; Vīrabhadrāsana I and II (9 and 10) for 10 seconds on each side; Pārśvottānāsana (13) for 10 seconds on each side; Prasārita Pādottānāsana (17) for 15 seconds; Uttānāsana (25) for 20 seconds; Sālamba Sarvāngāsana (102) for 5 minutes; Halāsana (113) for 5 minutes; Karṇapīdāsana (114) for 15 seconds; Suptakoṇāsana (115) for 15 seconds; Parśva Halāsana (116) for 15 seconds on each side; Ekapāda Sarvāngāsana (117) for 15 seconds on each side; Pārśvaikapāda Sarvāngāsana (118) for 15 seconds on each side; Setu Bandha Sarvāngāsana (121) for 1 minute; Ūrdhva Padmāsana and Pinḍāsana in Sarvāngāsana (122 and 123) for 15 seconds; Pārśva Pinḍāsana (124 and 125) for 15 seconds on each side; Jānu Śīrṣāsana (63); Ardha Baddha Padma Paschimottānāsana (66); Triang Mukhaikapāda Paschimottānāsana (69); Marīchyāsana I (71) all for 15 seconds on each side; Upaviṣṭha Koṇāsana (74) for 15 seconds; Paripūrṇa Nāvāsana (36) for 30 seconds; Ardha Nāvāsana (37) for 30 seconds; Baddha Koṇāsana (51) for 30 seconds; Paschimottānāsana (81) for 1 minute; Poorvottānāsana (82) for 15 seconds; Vīrāsana (42) and Supta Vīrāsana (49) for 15 seconds each; Parvatāsana in Padmāsana (54) for 30 seconds; Marichyāsana II (135 and 136) for 30 seconds on each side; Ardha Matyendrāsana (139 and 140) for 30 seconds on each side; Ūrdhva Dhanurāsana (114) for 3 times to capacity; Śavāsana (146) for 5 minutes. Nādi Śodhana Prāṇāyāma (Section 60) 8 cycles with inhalation retention. Dhyāna (150) for 3 minutes.

On Sundays do Nādi Śodhana Prāṇāyāma (Section 60) for 15 minutes with inhalation retention and Viloma Prāṇāyāma (Section 61) Stages I and II for 10 minutes in Śavāsana (146).

If one finds the number of āsanās or the length of time to do them has increased one can adjust according to capacity and the time at one's disposal.

Do Śavāsana (146) after Prāṇāyāma. Do Antarkumbhaka (inhalation retention) only when you have mastered the art of deep inhalation and deep exhalation without any jerks.

Do not do the āsanās and Prāṇāyāma together. You may feel strained and fatigued.

If you do Prāṇāyāma in the mornings then āsanās can be done in the evenings or half an hour after the āsanās.

Never do āsanās immediately after Prāṇāyāma, but one can practise Prāṇāyāma after āsanās if one is still fresh.

Those who wish to prostrate to the Sun (Sūryanamaskar) and to develop the arms and chest, can do the following āsanās in sequence at first for six rounds, increasing the number according to capacity.

	Āsanās	*Method of breathing*
1	Tāḍāsana (1)	Inhalation
2	Uttānāsana (25)	Exhalation, inhalation with head up
3	Chaturanga Danḍāsana (30)	Exhalation
4	Ūrdhva Mukha Svanasana (32) and go back to	Inhalation
5	Chaturanga Danḍāsana (30)	Exhalation, inhale
6	Adho Mukha Śvānāsana (33) and from here jump to	Exhale
7	Uttānāsana (25) and then back to	Inhalation
8	Tāḍāsana (1)	Exhalation

A Table to Correlate the Āsanas with the Plates that Illustrate them

Names of Āsanas, etc.	Intermediate Āsanas Plate No.	Final Āsanas Plate No.
1. Tāḍāsana	—	1
2. Utthita Trikoṇāsana	2	3 and 4
3. Utthita Pārśvakoṇāsana	—	5 and 6
4. Vīrabhadrāsana I	7 and 8	9
5. Virabhadrāsana II	—	10
6. Pārśvōttānāsana	11 and 12	13 and 14
7. Prasārita Pādottānāsana	15 and 16	17 and 18
8. Ustrāsana	19	20
9. Pādānguṣṭhāsana	21	22
10. Pāda Hastāsana	23	24
11. Uttānāsana	—	25
12. Śalabhāsana	27	26
13. Dhanurāsana	—	28
14. Chaturanga Daṇḍāsana	29	30
15. Bhujangāsana	—	31
16. Ūrdhva Mukha Śvānāsana	—	32
17. Adho Mukha Śvānāsana	—	33 and 34
18. Danḍāsana	—	35
19. Paripūrṇa Nāvāsana	—	36
20. Ardha Nāvāsana	—	37
21. Siddhāsana	—	38
22. Vīrāsana	39 to 41	42 to 45
23. Supta Vīrāsana	46 to 48	49
24. Baddha Koṇāsana	50	51 and 52
25. Padmāsana	—	53
26. Parvatāsana	—	54
27. Matsyāsana	55 and 57	56
28. Baddha Padmāsana	—	58 and 59
29. Yaga Mudrāsana	—	60
30. Mahā Mudrā	—	61
31. Jānu Śīrṣāsana	62	63

Names of Āsanas, etc.	Intermediate Āsanas Plate No.	Final Āsanas Plate No.
32. Ardha Baddha Padma Paschimottānāsana	64 and 65	66 and 67
33. Triang Mukhaikapāda Paschimottānāsana	68	69
34. Marīchyāsana I	70	71
35. Upaviṣṭha Koṇāsana	72 and 73	74
36. Paschimottānāsana (or Ugrāsana or Brahmacharyāsana)	75 to 80	81
37. Pūrvottānāsana	—	82
38. Sālamba Śīrṣāsana	83 to 89 and 92 to 95, 97	90, 91 and 96
39. Ūrdhva Daṇḍāsana	—	94
40. Sālamba Sarvāngāsana	98 to 101 and 104 to 107	102, 103 and 108
41. Halāsana	109 to 112	113
42. Karṇapīdāsana	—	114
43. Supta Koṇāsana	—	115
44. Pārśva Halāsana	—	116
45. Eka Pāda Sarvāngāsana	—	117
46. Pārśvaika Pāda Sarvāngāsana	—	118
47. Setu Bandha Sarvāngāsana (or Uttāna Mayūrāsana)	119 and 120	121
48. Ūrdhva Padmāsana in Sarvāngāsana	—	122
49. Pindāsana in Sarvāngāsana	—	123
50. Pārśva Piṇḍāsana in Sarvāngāsana	—	124 and 125
51. Jaṭhara Parivartanāsana	126	127 and 128
52. Supta Pādānguṣṭhāsana	129	130
53. Bharadvājāsana	—	131 and 132
54. Marīchyāsana II	133 and 134	135 and 136
55. Ardha Matsyendrāsana	137 and 138	139 and 140
56. Ūrdhva Dhanurāsana	141 to 143 and 145	144
57. Śavāsana	—	146
Prānāyāma		
58. Ujjāyi	—	147
59. Sūrya Bhedana	148	149
60. Nāḍi Śodhana	—	—
61. Viloma	—	—
— Dhyāna	—	150

Glossary

A	Negative particle meaning 'non', as in non-violence.
Abhaya	Freedom from fear.
Abhiniveśa	Instinctive clinging to life and the fear that one may be cut off from all by death.
Abhyāsa	Constant and determined study or practice.
Ādhaḥ	Down, lower.
Adhāra	A support.
Adhimātra	Beyond measure, superior.
Adhimātratama	The supreme one, the highest.
Adho-mukha	Face downwards.
Ādīśvara	The primeval Lord; an epithet of Śiva.
Advaita	Non-duality of the Universal Spirit with the individual soul.
Āgama	Testimony or proof of an acceptable authority when the source of knowledge has been checked and found trustworthy.
Ahaṁkāra	Ego or egotism; literally 'the I-Maker', the state that ascertains 'I know'.
Ahiṁsā	Non-violence. The word has not merely the negative and restrictive meaning of 'non-killing or non-violence', but the positive and comprehensive meaning of 'love embracing all creation'.
Ajapa-mantra	Unconscious repetitive prayer. Every living creature unconsciously breathes the prayer 'So'ham' (Saḥ=He (the Universal Spirit), aham=am I) with each inward breath, and with each outgoing breath prays 'Haṁsaḥ' (Aham=I am, Saḥ=He (the Universal Spirit)).
Akrodha	Freedom from anger.
Alabhdha-bhūmikatva	Failure to attain firm ground or continuity in practice, feeling that it is not possible to see reality.
Ālamba	Support.
Ālasya	Idleness, sloth, apathy.
Amanaska	The mind which is free from thoughts and desires.

Ananta	Infinite; a name of Viṣṇu as also of Viṣṇu's couch, the serpent Śeṣa.
Anavasthitattva	Instability to continue the practices feeling that it is not necessary to continue as he thinks that he has reached the highest state of Samādhi.
Aṅga	The body; a limb or a part of the body; a constituent part.
Aṅgamejayatva	Unsteadiness or tremor of the body.
Aṅgula	A finger; the thumb.
Aṅguṣṭha	The big toe.
Antara	Within; interior.
Antara Kumbhaka	Suspension of breath after full inhalation.
Antaranga Sādhanā	The inward quest of the soul by Prāṇāyāma and Pratyāhāra whereby the mind is brought under control and the senses are emancipated from the thraldom of objects of desire.
Antarātmā	The Supreme Soul residing in the heart of man.
Antarātmā Sādhanā	The innermost quest of the soul by means of Dhāranā (concentration), Dhyāna (meditation) and Samādhi.
Anumāna	An inference.
Apāna	One of the vital airs which move in the sphere of the lower abdomen and control the function of elimination of urine and faeces.
Aparigraha	Freedom from hoarding or collecting.
Apuṇya	Vice or demerit.
Ardha	Half.
Arjuna	A Pāṇḍava prince, the mighty bowman and hero of the epic Mahābhārata.
Āsana	Posture. The third stage of yoga.
Asmitā	Egotism.
Aṣṭa	Eight.
Aṣṭāṅga Yoga	The eight limbs of Yoga described by Patañjāli.
Asteya	Non-stealing.
Ātmā or *Ātman*	The Supreme Soul or Brahman.
Ātma Ṣaṭkam	A group of six verses written by Śankarāchārya describing the soul in the state of Samadhi.
Ātmīyatā	The feeling of oneness, as a mother's feeling for her children.
Auṁ	Like the Latin word 'Omne', the Sanskrit word 'Auṁ' means 'all' and conveys concepts of

	'Omniscience', 'Omnipresence' and 'Omnipotence'.
Avasthā	State or condition of the mind.
Avatāra	Descent, advent or incarnation of God. There are ten avatāras of Viṣṇu: Matsya (the Fish); Kūrma (the Tortoise); Varāha (the Boar), Narasiṁha (the Man-lion); Vāmana (the Dwarf); Paraśurāma; Rāma (hero of the epic Rāmāyaṇa); Krishna (hero of the epic Mahābhārata who related the Bhagavad Gīta); Balarāma and Kalki.
Avidyā	Ignorance.
Avirati	Sensuality.
Āyāma	Length, expansion, extension. It also conveys the idea of restraint, control and stopping.
Baddha	Bound, caught, restrained, firm.
Bahiraṅga Sādhanā	The outward quest of the soul for its Maker. The first three stages of Yoga, namely, Yama, Niyama and Āsana, are the outward quest and keep the seeker in harmony with his fellow men and nature.
Bāhya Kumbhaka	Suspension of breath after full exhalation when the lungs are completely empty.
Bandha	Bondage or fetter. It means a posture where certain organs or parts of the body are contracted and controlled.
Bhagavad Gītā	The Song Divine, the sacred dialogues between Krishna and Arjuna. It is one of the source books of Hindu philosophy, containing the essence of the Upanishads.
Bhagavān	Lord; venerable, holy.
Bhakti	Worship, adoration.
Bhakti-mārga	The way or path to realisation through adoration of a personal god.
Bharadvāja	A sage.
Bhaya	Fear.
Bhedana	Piercing, breaking through, passing through.
Bhoga	Enjoyment; an object of pleasure.
Bhoktṛ	One who enjoys or experiences.
Bhrānti-darśana	Erroneous (bhrānti) vision or knowledge (darśana), delusion.

Bhu	Land.
Bhūdāna	The donation of land.
Bhuja	The arm or the shoulder.
Bhujaṅga	A serpent, a snake.
Bhūmikatva	Firm ground.
Bīja	Seed or germ.
Bīja-mantra	A mystical syllable with a sacred prayer repeated mentally during prāṇāyāma, and the seed thus planted in the mind germinates into one-pointedness.
Brahmā	The Supreme Being, the Creator. The first deity of the Hindu Trinity entrusted with the work of creation of the world.
Brahma-vidyā	The knowledge of the Supreme Spirit.
Brahmachāri	A religious student vowed to celibacy and abstinence. One who is constantly moving (chārin) in Brahman (the Supreme Spirit); one who sees divinity in all.
Brahmacharya	A life of celibacy, religious study and self-restraint.
Brahman	The Supreme Being, the cause of the universe, the all-pervading spirit of the universe.
Brahmāṇḍa-prāṇa	The cosmic breath.
Buddhi	Intellect, reason, discrimination, judgement.
Chandra	The moon.
Chatur	The number four.
Chitta	The mind in its total or collective sense, being composed of three categories: (a) Mind, having the faculty of attention, selection and rejection; (b) Reason, the decisive state which determines the distinction between things and (c) Ego, the I-maker.
Chitta-vikṣepa	Distraction, confusion, perplexity.
Chitta-vṛtti	Fluctuations of the mind. A course of behaviour, mode of being, condition or mental state.
Dadhīcha	A celebrated sage, who donated his bones to the gods. From these bones was fashioned the thunderbolt, with which Indra, the king of the gods, slew the demon Vṛtra.

Dakṣa	A celebrated prajāpati, a lord of created beings.
Dakṣiṇa	The right side.
Damanī	A layer within a nāḍī or channel for the passage of energy.
Dānava	A demon.
Daṇḍa	A staff.
Daurmanasya	Despair, dejection.
Deva	A god.
Devadatta	One of the vital airs which provides for the intake of extra oxygen in a tired body by causing a yawn.
Dhanu	A bow.
Dhāraṇā	Concentration or complete attention. The sixth stage of Yoga mentioned by Patañjali.
Dhasaṁjaya	One of the vital airs which remains in the body even after death, and sometimes bloats up a corpse.
Dhṛ	To hold, to support, to maintain.
Dhyāna	Meditation. The seventh stage of Yoga mentioned by Patañjali.
Droṇa	The preceptor of the Pāṇḍava and Kaurava princes in the arts of war, especially archery. He was the son of the sage Bharadvāja.
Duḥkha	Pain, sorrow, grief.
Dveṣa	Hate, dislike, repugnance.
Dwi-hasta	Two hands.
Eka	One, single, alone, only.
Eka-tattvābhyāsa	The study of the single element, the Supreme Spirit that pervades the innermost self of all beings.
Ekāgra	(Ek=one; agra=foremost.) Fixed on one object or point only; closely attentive, where the mental faculties are all focused on a single object.
Ekāgratā	One-pointedness.
Gaṇa	A troop of demigods, who were Śiva's attendants.
Gaṅgā	The river Ganges, the most sacred river in India.
Gheraṇḍa	A sage, the author of Gheraṇḍa-Saṁhitā, a classical work on Haṭha-yoga.
Gheraṇḍa-Saṁhitā	*See* above.

Gu	First syllable in the word 'Guru', meaning darkness.
Gulma	The spleen.
Guṇa	A quality, an ingredient or constituent of nature.
Guṇātīta	One who is freed from and gone beyond or crossed the three guṇas of Sattva, Rajas and Tamas.
Guru	Spiritual preceptor, one who illumines the darkness of spiritual doubt.
Ha	First syllable of the word 'Haṭha', which is composed of the syllables 'ha' meaning the sun, and 'ṭha' meaning the moon. The object of Haṭha-yoga is to balance the flow of solar and lunar energy in the human system.
Hala	A plough.
'Haṁsaḥ'	'I am He, the Universal Spirit', the unconscious repetitive prayer that goes on with each exhalation within every living creature throughout life.
Hanumān	A powerful monkey chief of extraordinary strength and prowess, whose exploits are celebrated in the epic Rāmāyana. He was the son of Añjana and Vāyu, the god of wind.
Hasta	The hand.
Haṭha	Force. The word 'haṭha' is used adverbially in the sense of 'forcibly' or 'against one's will'. Haṭha-yoga is so called because it prescribes rigorous discipline, in order to find union with the Supreme.
Haṭha-vidyā	The science of Haṭha-yoga.
Haṭha-yoga	The way towards realisation through rigorous discipline.
Haṭha-yoga-pradīpikā	A celebrated textbook on Haṭha-yoga written by Svātmārāma.
Himālaya	The abode of ice and snow. Name of the mountain ranges on the northern borders of India.
Hiṁsā	Violence, killing.
Iḍā	A nāḍī, a channel of energy starting from the left nostril, then moving to the crown of the head and thence descending to the base of the spine.

	In its course it conveys lunar energy and so is called chandra nāḍī (channel of the lunar energy).
Indra	Chief of the gods. The god of thunder, lightning and rain.
Indriya	An organ of sense.
Indriya-jaya	Conquest, restraint or mastery of the senses by controlling desires.
Īśvara	The Supreme Being, God.
Īśvara-praṇidhāna	Dedication to the Lord of one's actions and one's will.
Jāgrata-avasthā	The complete awareness of the state of the mind.
Jālandhara-bandha	Jālandhara is a posture where the neck and throat are contracted and the chin is rested in the notch between the collar-bones at the top of the breast-bone.
Jamunā	A tributary of the Ganges.
Jānu	The knee.
Japa	A repetitive prayer.
Jatara-parivartana	An āsana, in which the abdomen is made to move to and fro.
Jaṭhara	The abdomen, stomach.
Jaya	Conquest, victory. It also means control, mastery.
Jīva	A living being, a creature.
Jīvana	Life.
Jīvana-mukta	A person who is emancipated during his lifetime by true knowledge of the Supreme Spirit.
Jīvana-mukti	The emancipated state.
Jīvātmā	The individual or personal soul.
Jñāna	Sacred knowledge derived from meditation on the higher truths of religion and philosophy, which teaches a man how to understand his own nature.
Jñāna-mārga	The path of knowledge by which man finds realisation.
Jñāna-mudrā	The gesture of the hand where the tip of the index finger is brought in contact with the tip of the thumb, while the remaining three fingers are kept extended. The gesture is a symbol of knowledge (jñāna). The index finger is the sym-

	bol of the individual soul, the thumb signifies the Supreme Universal Soul, and the union of these two symbolises true knowledge.
Jñānendriya	Hearing, touch, sight, taste and smell.
Kailāsa	A mountain peak in the Himālayas, considered as the abode of Śiva.
Kaivalya	Final emancipation.
Kaivalya-pāda	The fourth and last part of Patañjāli's Yoga Sūtra, dealing with Absolution.
Kālidāsa	The most renowned dramatist and poet in Sanskrit literature, whose work 'Śakuṅtalā' is universally respected.
Kapila	A sage, the founder of the Sānkhya system, one of the six orthodox systems of Hindu philosophy.
Karma	Action.
Karma-mārga	The way of an active man towards realisation through action.
Karma-yoga	The achievement of union with the Supreme Universal Soul through action.
Karmendriya	Organs of excretion, generation, hands, feet and speech.
Karṇa	The ear, also one of the heroes in the Mahābhārata.
Karṇa-pīdā	Pressure around the ear.
Karuṇā	Compassion, pity, tenderness. It also implies devoted action to alleviate the suffering of the afflicted ones.
Kaṭhopaniṣad	One of the principal Upanishads in verse and in the form of a dialogue between the seeker Nachiketā and Yama, the god of Death.
Kauravas	Descendants of Kuru, who fought the fratricidal Mahābhārata war with their cousins the Pāṇḍavas.
Kāyā	The body.
Kāyika	Relating to the body.
Kevala	Whole, entire, absolute, perfect, pure.
Kléśa	Pain, anguish, suffering.
Koṇa	An angle.
Krishṇa	The most celebrated hero in Hindu mythology. The eighth incarnation of Viṣṇu.

Kṛkara	Name of one of the subsidiary vital airs, whose function is to prevent substances going up the nasal passages and throat by bringing on sneezes and coughing.
Kṛta	Name of first of the four ages of the world of men.
Kṣatriya	A member of the warrior class.
Kṣipta	Distracted, neglected.
Kumbha	A water pot, a pitcher, a chalice.
Kumbhaka	Kumbhaka is the interval of time or retention of breath after full inhalation or after full exhalation.
Kuṇḍalinī	The Kuṇḍalinī (kuṇḍala=the coil of a rope; Kuṇḍalinī=a coiled female serpent) is the divine cosmic energy. This force or energy is symbolised as a coiled and sleeping serpent lying dormant in the lowest nerve centre at the base of the spinal column, the Mūlādhāra-chakra. This latent energy has to be aroused and made to ascend the main spinal channel, the Suṣumṇa piercing the chakras right up to the Sahasrāra, the thousand-petalled lotus in the head. Then the Yogi is in union with the Supreme Universal Soul.
Lac	100,000.
Laya	Dissolution; absorption of the mind, devotion.
Laya-yoga	The achievement of union with the Supreme Universal Soul through adoration or devotion.
Lobha	Greed.
Loma	Hair.
Madhyama	Middling, average, mediocre.
Mahā	Great, mighty, powerful, lofty, noble.
Mahābhārata	The celebrated epic composed by Vyāsa. It includes the Bhagavad Gītā.
Maharṣi	A great sage.
Maitri	Friendliness coupled with a feeling of oneness.
Man	To think.
Manas	The individual mind having the power and faculty of attention, selection and rejection. The ruler of the senses.

Manasika	Of the mind, mental.
Manomanī	The state of samādhi.
Mantra	A sacred thought or a prayer.
Manu	Name of the father of the human race.
Mārga	A way, road, path.
Marīchi	Name of one of the sons of Brahmā. He was a sage and the father of Kaśyapa, q.v.
Matsya	A fish.
Matsyendra	One of the founders of Haṭha-yoga.
Moha	Delusion, infatuation.
Mokṣa	Liberation, final emancipation of the soul from recurring births.
Mṛdu	Soft, gentle, mild.
Mṛta	Dead, a corpse.
Mūḍha	Perplexed, confounded, foolish, dull, stupid.
Muditā	Joy, delight.
Mudrā	A seal: a sealing posture.
Mukha	Face, mouth.
Mukta	Liberated.
Mukti	Release, liberation, final absolution of the soul from the chain of birth and death.
Muṇḍakopaniṣad	Name of a Upanishad dealing with the mystic syllable Auṁ.
Nachiketā	Name of the seeker and one of the principal characters in the Kaṭhopaniṣad. His father Vājaśravas wanted to give away all his possessions so as to acquire religious merit. Nachiketā felt puzzled and asked his father again and again: 'To whom will you give me?' His father said: 'I give you to Yama (the god of Death).' Nachiketā went down to the realm of Death and obtained three boons, the last of which was the knowledge of the secret of life after death. Yama tried to divert Nachiketā from obtaining his wish by offering the greatest earthly pleasures, but Nachiketā was not swayed from his purpose and ultimately Yama gave him the knowledge desired.
Nāda	Inner mystical sound.
Nāḍī	A tubular organ of the subtle body through which energy flows. It consists of three layers,

	one inside the other, like insulation of an electric wire. The innermost layer is called the 'sirā' and the middle layer 'damanī'. The entire organ as well as the outer layer is called 'nāḍī'.
Nāḍī-śodhana	The purification or cleansing of the nāḍīs.
Nāga	One of the subsidiary vital airs which relieves abdominal pressure, causing one to belch.
Nāva	A boat.
'Neti Neti'	'Not This! Not this!' The experience of samādhi is not like other experiences, which can be described in words. About it the sages say 'It is not this! It is not this!', for speech fails to convey the feeling of joy and peace experienced in that state.
Nirālamba	Without support.
Niranjana	Unstained; free from falsehood, pure.
Nirodha	Restraint, suppression.
Niruddha	Restrained, checked, controlled.
Niyama	Self-purification by discipline. The second stage of yoga mentioned by Patañjāli.
Pāda	The foot or leg; also part of a book.
Pādāṅguṣṭha	The big toe.
Padma	A lotus.
Pāṇḍava	Name of any of the five sons of Pāṇḍu, the heroes in the Mahābhārata.
Paramapāda	The highest step, the supreme state, final beatitude.
Paramātmā	The Supreme Spirit.
Parigraha	Hoarding.
Paripūrṇa	Entire, complete.
Parivartana	Turning round, revolving.
Parivṛtta	Turned around, revolved.
Parivṛttaika-pāda	With one leg turned around.
Pārśva	The side, flank; lateral.
Parśvaika-pāda	With one leg turned sideways.
Parvata	A mountain.
Pārvati	A goddess, consort of Śiva, daughter of Himālaya.
Paśchima	West; the back of the whole body from head to heels.

Paśchimottana	Intense stretch of the back side of the body from the nape to the heels.
Patañjali	The propounder of Yoga philosophy. He was the author of the Yoga Sūtras, the Mahābhāśya (a classical treatise on grammar) and a treatise on medicine.
Pīḍā	Pain, suffering, pressure.
Piṇḍa	The foetus or embryo, the body.
Piṇḍa-prāṇa	The individual breath, as contrasted with the cosmic or Universal breath.
Piṅgalā	A nāḍī or channel of energy, starting from the right nostril, then moving to the crown of the head and thence downwards to the base of the spine. As the solar energy flows through it it is also called the sūrya-nāḍī. Piṅgalā means tawny or reddish.
Plīhā	The spleen.
Prajñā	Intelligence, wisdom.
Prajñātmā	The intelligential self.
Prakṛti	Nature, the original source of the material world, consisting of three qualities, sattva, rajas and tamas.
Pramāda	Indifference, insensibility.
Pramāṇa	A standard or ideal; authority.
Prāṇa	Breath, respiration, life, vitality, wind, energy, strength. It also connotes the soul.
Prāṇa-vāyu	The vital air which pervades the entire human body. It moves in the region of the chest.
Praṇava	Another word for the sacred syllable Auṁ.
Prāṇāyāma	Rhythmic control of breath. The fourth stage of yoga.
Praṇidhāna	Dedication.
Prasārita	Spread out, stretched out.
Praśvāsa	Expiration.
Pratyāhāra	Withdrawal and emancipation of the mind from the domination of the senses and sensual objects. The fifth stage of yoga.
Pratyakṣa	Direct evidence.
Puṇya	Virtue, merit, righteous, just, good.
Puraka	Inhalation.
Pūrṇatā	Fullness, perfection.
Pūrva	East. The front of the body.

Pūrvottana	The intense stretch of the front side of the body.
Rāga	Love, passion, anger.
Rāja	A king, a ruler.
Rāja-mārga	The royal road to self-realisation through the control of the mind.
Rāja-yoga	The achievement of union with the Supreme Universal Spirit, by becoming the ruler of one's own mind by defeating its enemies. The chief of these enemies are: Kāma (passion or lust), krodha (anger or wrath), lobha (greed), moha (delusion), mada (pride) and matsara (jealousy or envy). The eightfold yoga of Patañjāli shows the royal road (rāja-mārga) for achieving this objective.
Rāja-yogī	One who has complete mastery over his mind and self. One who has conquered himself.
Rajas	Mobility or activity; one of the three qualities or constituents of everything in nature.
Rajo-guṇa	The quality of mobility or activity.
Rechaka	Exhalation, emptying of the lungs.
Ṛṣi	An inspired sage.
Ṛu	The second syllable in the word 'guru', meaning light.
Sādhaka	A seeker, an aspirant.
Sādhanā	Practice, quest.
Sādhana-pāda	The second part of Patañjāli's Yoga Sūtras, dealing with the means.
Sahajāvasthā	The natural state of the soul in samādhi.
Śalabha	A locust.
Sālamba	With support.
Sama	Same, equal, even, upright.
Sama-sthiti	Standing still and straight.
Samādhi	A state in which the aspirant is one with the object of his meditation, the Supreme Spirit pervading the universe, where there is a feeling of unutterable joy and peace.
Samādhi-pāda	The first part of Patañjali's Yoga Sūtras, dealing with the state of samādhi.
Samāna	One of the vital airs, whose function is to aid digestion.

Saṁśaya	Doubt.
Saṁskāra	Mental impression of the past.
Śankarāchārya	A celebrated teacher of the doctrine of Advaita.
Ṣaṇmukhī-mudrā	A sealing posture where the apertures in the head are closed and the mind is directed inwards to train it for meditation.
Santoṣa	Contentment.
Saraswatī	A tributary of the Ganges. Also the name of the goddess of speech and learning, the consort of Brahmā.
Sarva	All, whole.
Sarvāṅga	The whole body.
Satī	The daughter of Dakṣa Prajāpati. She immolated herself for the insult offered to her husband Śiva by her father, and was then reborn as the daughter of Himālaya and again won Siva as her husband. She was the mother of Kārtikeya (the god of war) and of Ganapati (the god of learning, wisdom and good luck).
Sattva	The illuminating, pure and good quality of everything in nature.
Sattva-guṇa	The quality of goodness and purity.
Śaucha	Purity, cleanliness.
Śava	A corpse, a dead body.
Setu	A bridge.
Setu-bandha	The construction of a bridge. Name of an āşana in which the body is arched.
Siddha	A sage, seer or prophet; also a semi-divine being of great purity and holiness.
Sirā	A tubular organ in the body. *See* nāḍī.
Śirṣa	The head.
Śiṣya	A pupil, a disciple.
Śiva	Name of the third god of the Hindu Trinity, who is entrusted with the task of destruction.
Śiva-saṁhitā	A classical textbook on Haṭha-yoga.
Smrti	Memory, a code of law.
Śodhana	Purification, cleansing.
'Soham'	'He am I'; the unconscious repetitive prayer that goes on with every inhalation within every living creature throughout life.
Śoka	Anguish, distress, grief, sorrow.
Śraddhā	Faith, trust.

Steya	Theft, robbery.
Sthita-prajñā	One whose wisdom is firmly established and does not waver; one who is unmoved by the dualities of pleasure and pain, gain and loss, joy and sorrow, victory and defeat.
Sthiti	Stability.
Styāna	Languor, sloth.
Sukha	Happiness, delight, joy, pleasure, comfort.
Sumanasya	Benevolence.
Śunyāśūnya	The mind is in a state of void (Śūnya) and yet a state that is not void (aśūnya).
Supta	Sleeping.
Sūrya	The sun.
Sūrya-bhedana	Piercing or passing through (bhedana) the sun. Here the inhalation is done through the right nostril, from where the Piṅgalā-nāḍī or Sūrya-nāḍī starts. Exhalation is done through the left nostril, from where the Iḍā-nāḍī or Chandra-nādī starts.
Sūrya-nāḍī	The nāḍī of the sun. Another name for Piṅgalā-nāḍī
Suṣumṇā	The main channel situated inside the spinal column.
Suṣupti-avasthā	The state of the mind in dreamless sleep.
Sva	One's own, innate, vital force, soul, self.
Svādhyāya	Education of the self by study of divine literature.
Śvāna	A dog.
Svapnāvasthā	The state of the mind in a dream.
Śvāsa	Inspiration.
Śvāsa-praśvāsa	Heaving and sighing.
Svātmārāma	The author of the Haṭha-yoga-pradīpikā, a classical textbook on Haṭha-yoga.
Tāḍa	A mountain.
Tamas	Darkness or ignorance, one of the three qualities or constituents of everything in nature.
Tamo-guṇa	The quality of darkness or ignorance.
Tan or *Tān*	To stretch, extend, lengthen out.
Tap	To burn, to blaze, to shine, to suffer pain, to be consumed by heat.

Tapas — A burning effort which involves purification, self-discipline and austerity.

'Tat twam asi' — 'That thou art.' The realisation of the real nature of man as being part of the divine, and of the divinity within himself, which liberates the human spirit from the confines of his body, mind, intellect and ego.

Tattva — The true or first principle, an element or primary substance. The real nature of the human soul or the material world and the Supreme Universal Spirit pervading the universe.

Tattva-jñāna — The knowledge of the true principle.

Tejas — Lustre, brilliance, majesty.

Ṭha — The second syllable of the word 'haṭha'. The first syllable 'ha' stands for the sun, while the second syllable 'ṭha' stands for the moon. The union of these two is Haṭha-yoga.

Tirieng — Horizontal, oblique, transverse, reverse and upside down.

Tri — Three.

Triaṅga — Three limbs.

Trikoṇa — A triangle.

Tṛṣṇā — Thirst, longing, desire.

Turīyāvasthā — The fourth state of the soul, combining yet transcending the other three states of waking, dreaming and sleeping state – the state of samādhi.

Ubhaya — Both.

Udāna — One of the vital airs which pervades the human body, filling it with vital energy. It dwells in the thoracic cavity and controls the intake of air and food.

Ugra — Formidable, powerful, noble.

Ujjāyi — A type of prāṇāyāma in which the lungs are fully expanded and the chest is puffed out.

Unmanī — The state of samādhi.

Upaniṣad — The word is derived from the prefixes 'upa' (near) and 'ni' (down), added to the root 'sad' (to sit). It means sitting down near a Guru to receive spiritual instruction. The Upanishads are the philosophical portion of the Vedas, the most ancient sacred literature of the Hindus, dealing with the nature of man and the universe and the union of the individual soul or self with the Universal Soul.

Upaviṣṭha — Seated.

Upekṣā — Disregard. Upekṣā is not only a feeling of disdain for a person who has fallen into vice or a feeling of indifference or superiority towards him. It is also a self-examination to find out how one would have behaved in like circumstances and also how far he is responsible for the state of the fallen one and to help him on to the right path.

Ūrdhva — Raised, elevated, tending upwards.

Ūrdhva-mukha — Face upwards.

Uṣṭra — A camel.

Ut — A particle, denoting intensity.

Uttāna — An intense stretch.

Utthita — Raised up, extended, stretched.

Vāchā — Speech.

Vāchika — Relating to speech, oral.

Vairāgya — Absence of worldly desires.

Vajra — A thunderbolt, the weapon of Indra.

Valli — A chapter of the Upanishads.

Vāma — The left side.

Vāsanā — Desire, inclination, longing.

Vasiṣṭha — A celebrated sage, author of several Vedic hymns.

Vāyu — The wind, the vital airs.

Veda — The sacred scriptures of the Hindus, revealed by the Supreme Being.

Vibhūti — Might, power, greatness.

Vibhūti-pāda — The third part of the Yoga Sūtras of Patañjāli, dealing with the powers that the yogi comes across in his quest.

Vidyā — Knowledge, learning, lore, science.

Vikalpa — Fancy, resting merely on verbal expression, without any factual basis.

Vikṣepa — Distraction, confusion, perplexity.

Vikṣipta — Agitated state of the mind.

Viloma	Against the hair, against the order of things. The particle 'vi' denotes negation or privation.
Viparyaya	A mistaken view, which is later observed to be such, after study.
Vīra	A hero, brave.
Vīrabhadra	A powerful hero created out of Śiva's matted hair.
Virochana	A demon prince, who was the son of Prahlāda and the father of Bali.
Vīrya	Vigour, strength, virility, enthusiasm.
Viṣama-vṛtti	Uneven or vehement movement while breathing.
Viṣṇu	The second deity of the Hindu trinity, entrusted with the preservation of the world.
Viśvāmitra	A celebrated sage.
Vitasti	A span.
Vṛkṣa	A tree.
Vṛt	To turn, to revolve, to roll on.
Vṛtti	A course of action, behaviour, mode of being, condition or mental state.
Vyādhi	Sickness, disease, illness.
Vyāna	One of the vital airs, which pervades the entire body and circulates the energy derived from food and breathing all over the body.
Yama	The god of death. Yama is also the first of the eight limbs or means of attaining yoga. Yamas are universal moral commandments or ethical disciplines transcending creeds, countries, age and time. The five mentioned by Patañjali are: non-violence, truth, non-stealing, continence and non-coveting.
Yoga	Union, communion. The word 'yoga' is derived from the root 'yuj' meaning to join, to yoke, to concentrate one's attention on. It is the union of our will to the will of God, a poise of the soul which enables one to look evenly at life in all its aspects. The chief aim of yoga is to teach the means by which the human soul may be completely united with the Supreme Spirit pervading the universe and thus secure absolution.
Yoga-mudrā	A posture.

Yoga Sūtra — The classical work on yoga by Patañjali. It consists of 185 terse aphorisms on yoga and it is divided into four parts dealing respectively with samādhi, the means by which yoga is attained, the powers the seeker comes across in his quest and the state of absolution.

Yogi or *Yogin* — One who follows the path of yoga.

Yoni-mudrā — Yoni means the womb or source and mudrā a seal. Yoni-mudrā is a sealing posture where the apertures of the head are closed and the aspirant's senses are directed within to enable him to find out the source of his being.

Yuga — An age.

Yuj — To join, to yoke, to use, to concentrate one's attention on.

Yukta — One who has attained communion with the Supreme Spirit pervading the universe.

Index